AF443596

RISK IN SOCIETY

Risk in society is based on the First International Risk Seminar held at the Royal College of Physicians (by kind permission of the Treasurer) under the Patronage of Lord Zuckerman, London, March 1983, sponsored by Information TRANSFER International. Further seminars will be published in the series *International Monographs on Risk*.

International Monographs on Risk
(ISSN 0266-0512)

1:   Risk in society ed A J Jouhar ISBN 0 86196 034 3
2:   Modelling and simulation for safety and risk assessment ed A J Jouhar ISBN 0 86196 041 6

RISK IN SOCIETY

Proceedings of the
First International Risk Seminar

Editor
A J JOUHAR

Foreword by
LORD ZUCKERMAN OM KCB FRS

John Libbey: London and Paris

British Library cataloguing in publication data

International Risk Seminar *(1st: 1983: Royal College of Physicians)*
    Risk in society. — (International monographs on risk, ISSN 0266 - 0512)
    1. Risk management
    I. Title II. Jouhar, A.J. III. Series
    658.4'03 HD61

    ISBN 0 - 86196 - 034 - 3

First published 1984 by
John Libbey & Company Limited
80-84 Bondway, London SW8 1SF, England
6 rue Blanche, 92120 Montrouge, France
© 1984 Copyright
All rights reserved

Printed in Great Britain by Whitstable Litho Ltd, Whitstable, Kent

FOREWORD

by

LORD ZUCKERMAN OM KCB FRS

In days gone by it was very unusual for concern to be expressed about public hazards before they had revealed themselves, before, for example, water supplies had become polluted, or before the customer had been sold adulterated food. Public health laws were then enacted on the basis of whatever hard experience was available. When typhoid struck, contacts had to be traced to discover the source - as indeed remains the case today. It was not until 1976 that we had an Act of Parliament which legitimised spot checks on the cleanliness of kitchens and restaurants that cater to the public. When I was a medical student in the 1920s the pharmacopoeia of my teaching hospital still listed as a standard remedy for intestinal upsets lead and opium pills; and that, remarkably enough, at a time when it was already known that lead in sufficient dose is a poison. Maybe my medical school was a bit out of date. As early as the latter part of the 17th century, the adulteration of wine with Sapa, a sweet syrup with a high lead content, had been declared a capital offence in the State of Wurtemburg. Obviously it would have been impossible in those days to enforce the law by making check analyses on the wine that was offered for sale. Nor was it the purpose of the law to provide some form of compensation or redress for those who had already been poisoned. The law was there to deter would-be malefactors.

The succession of the UK's Food and Drug Acts, beginning with that of 1875, have had the same deterrent purpose - to protect the citizen against being cheated and from being harmed by dangerous food additives and drugs. As I have already said, early laws were based on such facts as were available at the time. Today, when there is no real evidence to which to turn, we have regulations that demand that new food additives, new drugs or new agrochemicals be rigorously tested in the laboratory before they can be licensed for sale. We not only have our own laws but, in the interests of international trade, we also have to conform to internationally agreed test procedures. But, as we know to our cost, despite all precautionary measures accidents still happen.

The public's ever-increasing awareness of what is going on in our changing world makes it inevitable that efforts to undertake 'risk assessments' - by which is meant the conscious effort to measure the nature and scale of possible hazards - are with us to stay. They have to be made in an environment composed of all gradations of ignorance and fear. However remote the possibility that there ever will be a tidal surge in the North Sea on a scale sufficient to pour millions of tons of water over the banks of the Thames, a barrage has had to be built at enormous cost lest thousands of Londoners be one day drowned. Probability calculations have been made of the likelihood of this kind of hazard as they have been of a disaster in a nuclear power plant. The public is concerned about these hazards; others, equally remote, are disregarded, such as, for example, the possibility that the consequences of acid rain could imperil the total environment to which mankind is now adapted. There may be other hazards that now defy the imagination, but which could turn out to be real.

But the problem is not just that of making academic assessments of degrees of risk. As important - perhaps even more important - is the tax-payer's reaction to measures to deal with risks, and the state's ability to find the resources to make measures effective. The public will accept the need for general vaccination against some plague when it recognises that every one of us would be better off were it the case - as it has been in that of smallpox and diptheria - that the disease could be eradicated. On the other hand, many prefer to believe that the pleasures of smoking outweigh the risk that lung cancer may be one of its consequences. In such cases, the state cannot move, mainly because it needs the consent of the people to act. And when it comes to such matters as dealing with the atmospheric pollution that results from the burning of fossil fuels, it might well be that effective action will go on being deferred because of the lack of the very resources which derive from the sale of the goods that are turned out by the manufacturing plants which are responsible for the pollution. What needs to be borne in mind is the possibility that the day may come when the consequences of not dealing with such seemingly remote problems as acid rain become very much more serious than would be those of finding the resources to deal with fossil fuel burners today.

It is because we are becoming increasingly conscious of the precarious environment in which we live that sophisticated risk analyses have become the order of the day, and risk seminars such as the one recorded in this volume so valuable. Forewarned is forearmed. There is no point in terrifying ourselves with groundless fears; there is point in understanding when fear is justified. What we want is more of the kind of knowledge which tells where the balance of risk lies.

9 August 1983

University of East Anglia
Norwich, England

PREFACE

This book records the proceedings of the First International Risk Seminar which took place at the Royal College of Physicians in London (by kind permission of the Treasurer) on 14 and 15 March, 1983.

The Seminar was conceived as an attempt to review the diverse opinions held by those in differing disciplines on hazards, associated risks and the acceptability of risk, with particular reference to chemicals. Invited contributors were asked to consider the following questions:

1. What are the hazards and risk levels that exist in society today; what are the risks to the consumer and to the industrial worker from chemicals and what views are taken by industry? Are there special problems for the elderly and what does society do about this? Can we relate short and long-term hazards in assessing risk?

2. Dealing further with the interaction of chemicals and people, what can we learn from morbidity and mortality statistics; what particular problems are there with therapeutic chemicals and with those used in consumer goods, in the risk-benefit equation? Can we extrapolate hazard and risk from experimental data?

3. Does the 'acceptable risk' exist? How is this concept seen from historical data; is there biological justification; how does society perceive differing risks; what are societal/governmental attitudes to accepting risk levels; can we 'scale' the human effects of health hazards?

From the list of contributors and their subjects, the reader will see that a multi-disciplinary approach was taken in dealing with these questions. It was clear from the outset that no agreement would be reached. The value of such a Seminar - and for the reader of the Proceedings - lies in assessing the bases for the variety of opinions on the emotive concept captured by the phrase 'one man's meat is another's poison'.

Put another way, '*your* risk may be for *my* benefit and what *I* can accept on *your* behalf may not be acceptable to *you* - but *I* think *you* should accept it anyway! (or the converse)'.

The book is divided into four parts; the first and second deal with risks in society and risks from chemicals, respectively. The third and fourth focus on the concept of the acceptable risk and the implications of this concept for society and for government.

The sponsors for this Seminar, Information TRANSFER International, express their gratitude to Lord Zuckerman OM KCB FRS for so readily agreeing to be Patron; to the Chairmen for the various sections of the Seminar; and to the other contributors. Due to pressure of work, it was not possible for two contributors to the Seminar (Mr Tam Dalyell, MP and Professor Lee) to provide papers for inclusion in these Proceedings.

1983   A J Jouhar

SEMINAR CHAIRMEN

Dr William W Lowrance, Senior Fellow and Director, Life Sciences and Public Policy Program, The Rockefeller University, 1230 York Avenue, New York NY 10021, USA.

Professor Terence R Lee, Department of Psychology, University of Surrey, Guildford, Surrey GU2 5XH, England.

Dr Robert P Giovacchini, VP Corporate Product Integrity, The Gillette Company, 1413 Research Boulevard, Rockville, Maryland 20850, USA.

Dr Jan Jouhar, Consultant in Human Biological Affairs and Chief Executive - Information TRANSFER International, PO Box 62, Beaconsfield, Bucks HP9 2NY England.

SEMINAR CONTRIBUTORS

Dr William W Lowrance, Senior Fellow and Director, Life Sciences and Public Policy Program, The Rockefeller University, 1230 York Avenue, New York NY 10021, USA.

Dr Lesley Yeomans, Research Manager, Consumers' Association, 14 Buckingham Street, London WC2N 6DS, England.

Dr R F Griffiths, Assistant Director, Pollution Research Unit, The University of Manchester Institute of Science & Technology, PO Box 88, Manchester M60 1QD, England.

Professor P H Millard, Department of Geriatric Medicine, St George's Hospital, Clare House, Blackshaw Road, London SW17 0QT, England.

Professor Trevor Kletz, 40 Hall Drive, Acklam, Middlesborough, Cleveland TS5 7ET, England.

Professor Terence R Lee, Department of Psychology, University of Surrey, Guildford, Surrey GU2 5XH, England.

Dr Roy Goulding, Consultant, 36 Ashley Court, Morpeth Terrace, London SW1P 1EN, England.

Professor M F Oliver, Cardiovascular Research Unit, Hugh Robson Building, George Square, Edinburgh EH8 9XF, Scotland.

M.J Collin, Commission of the European Communities-DGXI, Rue de la Loi 200, B - 1049 Brussels, Belgium.

Dr Francis J C Roe, Consultant, 19 Marryat Road, Wimbledon Common, London SW19 5B, England.

Dr Robert P Giovacchini, VP Corporate Product Integrity, The Gillette Company, 1413 Research Boulevard, Rockville, Maryland 20850, USA.

Dr I F Carney, Central Toxicology Adviser, Imperial Chemical Industries, Alderley Park, Macclesfield, Cheshire SK10 4TJ, England.

Professor Jens S Schou, Department of Pharmacology, University of Copenhagen, 20 Juliane Mariesvej, DK-2100 Copenhagen 0, Denmark.

Dr Jack Dowie, Senior Lecturer in Social Science, The Open University, Walton Hall, Milton Keynes, MK7 6AA, England.

Clive Jenkins, General Secretary, ASTMS, 79 Camden Road, London NW1 9ES, England.

The Right Hon Tam Dalyell, Member of Parliament, House of Commons, Westminster, London SW1A 0AA, England.

Dr Robert J Scheuplein, Deputy Director of Toxicology, Bureau of Foods, Food and Drug Administration, 200 C Street, Washington 20204, USA.
Mme G Gobinet, Partial Agreements Public Health Division, Council of Europe, 67000 Strasbourg, France.
Dr Jan Jouhar, Consultant in Human Biological Affairs and Chief Executive - Information TRANSFER International, PO Box 62, Beaconsfield, Bucks HP9 2NY England

CONTENTS

Foreword **Lord Zuckerman OM KGB FRS** v

Preface vii

Contributors viii

PART 1 **RISK AND SOCIETY**

1 Improved science, heightened societal aspirations, and the agenda for 'risk' 3
  decision-making
  William W Lowrance

2 Risks to consumers 11
  Lesley Yeomans

3 Uncertainties in risk estimation and implications for risk management in industry 17
  R F Griffiths

4 Risk, age and society 27
  Peter H Millard

5 Now or later? A numerical comparison of short and long-term hazards 30
  Trevor Kletz

PART 2 **RISK FROM CHEMICALS**

6 Medical priorities - the place of chemicals 41
  Roy Goulding

7 Risk of correcting risks of cardiovascular disease by drugs 48
  Michael F Oliver

8 Hazards and risk levels associated with consumer goods 51
  Jean Collin

9 Extrapolation of risk from low-potency animal carcinogens 55
  Francis J C Roe

PART 3 **THE ACCEPTABLE RISK - DOES IT EXIST?**

10 An overview of the problem 67
  Robert P Giovacchini

11 The empirical approach : vinyl chloride - a cancer case study 73
  Ian F Carney

12 Biological considerations 78
  Jens S Schou

13 Perceived risk: a chimera? 83
  Jack Dowie

14 Risk assessment and the control of toxic substances in the work place 94
  Clive Jenkins

PART 4 **SOCIETAL IMPLICATIONS & GOVERNMENTAL ATTITUDES**

15 Regulation of low-level carcinogenic risk in foods: the United States view 111
Robert J Scheuplein

16 The acceptable risk and the Council of Europe 117
Gilly Gobinet

17 'Scaling' human effects from physico-chemical hazards 120
A J Jouhar

INDEX 127

PART 1

Risk And Society

1

Improved science, heightened societal aspirations and the agenda for 'risk' decision-making

WILLIAM W LOWRANCE

The keynote I would strike for this meeting is, that :

The extraordinary current improvements in science, coming into conjunction with heightened societal aspirations, will strongly influence society's decision-making.

Experience in the past decade with such issues as saccharin, polio vaccination, space exploration, contraception, and energy policy has brought broad public recognition of the lessons that nothing can be risk-free, that there are no rewards without risks, and that risk taking for benefit is the essence of human striving.

'Risk' generally has come to mean a factual estimate of the likelihood and severity of deleterious effect. Societal or personal decisions about sources of risk are then understood to be appraisive, taking into account such considerations as benefits, costs, equities, and political dynamics, as well as risks. At issue may be whether a particular risk is 'acceptable', or as low as is reasonably achievable, or is similar to risks already accepted or to the risks of alternatives. It has become clear that empirical estimates of risk are value-conditioned (as all questioning is) and that facts can be generated about people's values.

Now, at least in the United States, one rarely hears demands anymore for 'zero risk', even from the Congress, and courts no longer declaim that 'Human life is beyond all price....', which never did mean anything. We are putting firmer reins on some technologies, such as nuclear reactors, whose technical development simply outran society's management. And we are cleaning up some messy legacies, such as those of asbestos and toxic waste, about which both our scientific understanding and our values have changed. We have become more restrained in releasing materials into the environment. We have redefined 'environment' to include not just outdoors but also workplaces, schools, and homes. And we have become more cautious about taking irreversible actions.

"

Threats, however, continue to proliferate. Recent additions to the apprehension-list include marijuana smoke, textile dust, wood dust, formaldehyde, indoor radon, video display screens, low-frequency elect romagnetic radiation from direct-current powerlines, genital herpes, toxic shock syndrome, Acquired Immune Deficiency Syndrome, industrial lasers, robotic tools, acid rain.... New automobiles, tools, toys, and chemicals will always come along. All of these need attention; some will prove harmless, some will need controlling.

What of the broad-scope agenda?

Maturation of society's outlook on risk issues must be the pervasive theme. Two attitudinal changes are essential, if we are to avoid being overwhelmed emotionally and procedurally by all the emergencies, warnings, false alarms, and controversies: we must come to terms with the essentially tragic nature of these matters, and we must learn to view risk-management actions as societal investments.

What is crucial is to recognize that, as with other aspects of modernity, mankind's confrontation of risks to health and well-being has become deeply tragic: we now experience *tragic awarenesses* of risks and their causes, we have to make *tragic choices* among life-expensive goals, and we must bear *tragic commitments* to the consequences of our choices.

By 'tragic' I don't mean merely unhappy, but rather (with Whitehead) a sense of the 'solemnity of the remorseless working of things', especially as human will intervenes. By describing flatly *the way things are,* science raises tragic awarenesses about events, causes, and human agency; intentionality displaces 'blind chance', and odds and stakes become subject to deliberate alteration. In making tragic choices we must choose among near-irreconcilable goals, with at least some foreknowledge of the likely consequences of our decisions. And tragically we must commit ourselves to the futures chosen, as in protecting deposits of high-level radioactive waste, dealing with the results of genetic engineering, and maintaining the Netherlands dykes, These awarenesses, choices, and commitments may leave us happy or not; but of their solemnity there can be no question.

Certainly health in the industrial West is, in general, more robust than ever before. We have conquered some of the most dangerous infectious diseases, such as tuberculosis, diphtheria, smallpox, cholera, typhus, and polio, and we have made progress against many others. Scurvy, pellagra, iron-deficiency anaemia, and other nutritional diseases have been mastered. Many illnesses that have not yet been eliminated, such as diabetes, have at least been brought under control. Exposure to mercury, lead, arsenic, chromium, and other heavy-metal poisons has been sub-stantially reduced, as has exposure to asbestos, halocarbon solvents, and many other chemicals. Through prediction and protection, damage from storms and earthquakes has been mitigated. Overall, infant mortality continues to decrease, and life expectancy increase. More people are living longer, healthier, more vigorous lives.

Nonetheless, almost ruefully, we have progressed to an inherently discomfiting state, a state in which we must expect to remain.

Why inherently discomfiting? Because steadily we have broadened our risk concerns to include not only natural catastrophes, infectious diseases, everyday mechanical accidents, and acute poisons, but also large-scale technological accidents, chronic low-level hazards from chemicals, radiation, and noise, and even 'life-style' vices, such as addictions to tobacco, alcohol, barbiturates, hard drugs, caffeine, and overeating. To our struggle against classical scourges we have added concern about reproductive genetic, immunological, behavioural, and other debilitations. And of course we continue to create new hazards, to identify risks that may have been present but not recognized, and to resolve to reduce various risks that we have long tolerated.

Now, about many hazards we know enough, scientifically, to 'worry', but not enough to know *how much* to worry - or how much protective action to invest. Scientific knowledge has progressed enormously, and we even have the luxury of going around searching for possible trouble. But many scientific disciplines are still in their adolescence and are unable to evaluate risks precisely. (We can detect miniscule traces of manmade chlorocarbons in mothers' milk all over the world, which is vaguely disturbing, but we don't have a clue as to whether the chemicals exert any effect on mother or infant.) Investigative medicine, toxicology, epidemiology, and engineering analysis have taken us out to their borders; but it's unruly territory.

Part of the problem is that risks evolve. In his 1803 *Essay on Population* Thomas Malthus observed of Jenner's new vaccine, 'I have not the slightest doubt that if the introduction of cowpox should extirpate the smallpox, we shall find... increased mortality of some other disease'. Malthus was right. As any risk is reduced, others inevitably increase in the mortality and morbidity tables - though perhaps setting-in later in life. Risks are evolving now as rural and agrarian risks are succeeded by urban, industrial, and medical-care risks.

At the same time that we have been learning more about risks, we have been heightening our societal aspirations beyond all previous limits. We intend to help all infants get a vigorous start in life. And we strive to afford first-rate health protection (broadly defined) to all citizens, and even noncitizens, through an enormous range of risks, throughout their lives. No civilization ever before has had these ambitions.

The crux: In our knowing so much more and aspiring to so much more, we have passed beyond the sheltering blissfulness of ignorance and risk-enduring resignation. This has generated considerable social apprehensiveness, which is affecting both the outlook of individuals and the functioning of institutions.

Similar phase-changes have occurred historically when people became aware of specific causes of disease and deformity, as when it became clear that moral turpitude alone was not the cause of syphilis, and when societal aspirations, such as commitment to worker protection, rose. We are going through both kinds of changes at the same time.

One corrective against despair is to inculcate a view of risk-management efforts as societal investments - investments that yield returns in health costs saved, disruptions reduced, productivity enhanced. Another corrective is to build frameworks of perspective, within which new concerns can be appraised

The central methodological task is to develop ways of inter-comparing sources of risk, comparing risks against risks, weighing risks against the benefits they accompany, and appraising the societal return from reducing risks.

Comparative analysis can inform the setting of priorities, and thus help avoid frittering away worry-capital on very small hazards, help prohibit unbearably large hazards, and help concentrate on hazards in the middle range that affect many people in important ways, and that are susceptible to alteration.

Analysis can, for example, size up relative contributions to infant mortality, relative erosions of longevity, relative estimated mutagenic or cirrhotic potency, relative increment of insurance claims. Analysis can profile the frequency and severity of hazards, to indicate how likely catastrophic accidents are. Analysis can rank risks as to their tractability or cost-effectiveness of solution.

Sets within which risks can be compared include: *physical agents having definable effects* (radiation); *societal functions* (food preservation); *geographic area* (the Ruhr valley); *an industry* (glassmaking); *product class* (pest-control agents); *contributions to specified illness* (cirrhosis); or *contributions to mortality*.Analysis can indicate opportunities for risk research, reduction, redistribution, or compensation.

Such analyses provide perspective, reveal the relative 'payoff' of programmes, and help set defensible priorities. They are essential for determining which carcinogens, or toxic waste dumps, or consumer goods, or parts of a factory, deserve most attention. parts of a factory, deserve most attention.

Especially challenging in coming years will be comparative assessment of very large, complex technological systems. Attempts to survey the risks, benefits, and costs of nuclear power in comparison with those of fossil-fuel, hydropower, and other energy sources have shown how hard this is to do, especially if the assessment covers everything from fuel aquisition to waste disposal, from construction to eventual dismantlement, from mutagenesis to terrorism. The British experience in analyzing the risks to residents of the densely industrial Canvey Island, which helped identify opportunities for reducing the risks and planning Canvey's future, has been a most illuminating exercise. European and American analysis of the risks associated with the liquefied-natural-gas industry has been very helpful in choosing among options. We will be needing more of this kind of work, and we should draw lessons from these experiences.

A constructive but discomfiting aspect of all this is that our analyses and decisions are making us face risks ever more explicitly. The Health and Safety Executive compared Canvey residents' accidental death risks to those of other Britons, citing numbers. The US Food and Drug Administration has proposed to allow diethylstilbestrol (DES) feed-additive residues to remain in marketed beef at levels that might induce cancer in up to one-in-a-million consumers exposed over a lifetime, a risk the agency considers to be an insignificant addition to the hundreds and thousands of cases induced by smoking and other causes. The Environmental Protection Agency quantifies the estimated carcinogenic risk from pesticides it registers. Recently the Nuclear Regulatory Commission has promulgated safety goals that would hold powerplant-worker fatalities to no more than one death per thousand megawatts of electricity generated. Such candor is laudable - besides, risks can be calculated from the record even if authorities don't state them - but the explicitness is unsettling. Such knowledge raises tragic awareness.

Tragic choices inescapably will have to be confronted - not just made (we do that already), but confronted. We are straining our resources to the margins both in managing these environmental health risks and in providing expensive remedial medical care, such as renal dialysis. *We will not be able to afford everything for everybody.* The confrontation is coming.

A consequent challenge for the agenda is to work from these comparative assessments toward defining 'insignificant' or 'negligible' risk, 'acceptable' risk, and 'intolerable' or 'unacceptable' risk, and developing guidelines for decison. These notions cannot be derived from abstract principles but must be defined by debate and inferred from how people actually deal with risks.

We should *not* expect to arrive at precise and invariant demarcations, but at working-distinctions that can be re-evaluated at any time in the light of new knowledge or revised social values. For example, the US Food and Drug Administration has ruled the risks of several hairdyes and food-colourings 'insignificant' compared to other hazards, and the Environmental Protection Agency has banned commerce in polychlorinated biphenyls (PCBs) which it has deemed intolerably hazardous; either judgement could change.

Analysis usually does not consist of anything so crass as asking 'How much is one life worth?', but rather in asking such questions as 'What marginal investment in precaution will preserve marginally how many lives, or person-life-years, or eyes, from being lost to (some) hazard?', or,'Where can a given investment be most effective in protecting people?'.

Like the Zen query about the sound of one hand clapping, usually it doesn't make much sense to ask only about risks without enquiring about benefits and costs. Risk-levels that we might tolerate for some benefits, such as protection against fatal disease, we might well hold unacceptable if associated with, say, only cosmetic benefits.

We are going to have to admit that most of our decision frameworks really are only versions of one framework. Regulation-drafters often distinguish between 'absolute no risk' rules, benefit-risk balancing, cost-effectiveness, 'best available technological control', protection 'as low as is reasonably achievable', and the like. But, really, if actual implementation is considered, these are distinctions without differences: 'zero-risk' rules simply have been ignored when obeying them would be too costly for the benefit achieved; 'available' control and 'reasonable' achievability have been defined, analysis does not estimate benefits, it assumes the benefits to be worth the effectively-spent costs.

Throughout this conference we will be discussing how to compare instant deaths against delayed deaths (as in nuclear reactor decisions), 'bulked' harm against similar but diffuse harm (as in airliner standards compared to small-aircraft standards), intense hazard to a few people against smaller hazard to more (as in the rationing of nuclear workers' radiation exposure).

Another task for the agenda is to provide bases for reconciling non-expert popular opinions about risk issues with those of experts. This problem was exemplified a few years ago when Nobel biochemist Rosalyn Yalow wrote a *New York Times* 'op-ed' article (31 January 1981) about the closing of sites for disposal of low-level radioactive waste from biomedical reseach, in which she complained: 'The Nuclear Regulatory Commission should have proposed a change in regulations long before the sites were closed down. Why didn't it? The regulators were responding not to the *real* risk but rather to the public's fears of radiation at any level.... We must respond to real risk, not perception of risk.'

Such disputes strongly test republican forms of government, in which legitimated expert authorities are charged with making determinations on behalf of the public. They also entail a problematic distinction between 'subjective' and 'objective' opinions: all thinking is, by definition, 'subjective'; but questions such as what relative contribution different sources make to people's radioactivity exposure can, by scrutiny within the organized scepticism of science, become authenticated into knowledge that is reliable - knowledge that can describe and predict with consistency and accuracy *what is* and *what will happen* in the physical and biological world. While I reserve my right to evaluate the social importance of Dr Yalow's radwaste differently from the way she might, I also protest that I don't want my radiation protection determined by public-opinion polls! (Parenthetically I hasten to say, also, that I object to the arrogant term 'real risk'; one persons's objectivity is another's subjectivity, and, in science as elsewhere, many value biases influence construction of 'the real'.) Comparisons, and the exercise of making them, can help resolve differences in views.

Psychologists are studying how people perceive risks, and decision theorists are developing typologies of values and valuation processes. I am sceptical of much of this work, which I find simplistic. Few of its results have found application in policy design or decision-making. Opinion polls that don't force respondents to make tradeoffs are not very revealing. Too, perceptions are subject to rapid shifts: hydropower will probably continue to be viewed as harmless, until the day a large dam breaks over a major population centre.

We do need better mechanisms for soliciting and responding to the public's (or, various publics') opinions. Risk-management regimens must strive to make just and efficient investment of resources. But they also must evaluate the public's preferences and allay public apprehensions and the instabilities they induce. This latter function should not be understated, as some deposed American government officials would testify. Inversely, on issues such as fluoridation of drinking water, vaccination against polio, or regulation of automobile safety, we need better ways of communicating experts' evaluations to the public.

Much can be learned by studying people's willingness to pay for hazard reduction, adopt protective measures, choose among medical therapeutic options, insure themselves and others against loss, and compensate those who incur harm from occupational exposure or natural disaster.

Looking toward the future, the agenda must become more self-reflexive, to anticipate demographic and hazard apprehension changes. As our populations age, the spectrum of illnesses changes. Degenerative illnesses, such as heart disease and cancer, of course have been increasing (although these two may now be plateauing). In addition to acutely fatal illnesses, concern is growing over long-term debilitations, such as arthritis, hayfever, and cirrhosis, and over a variety of renal, neurological, endocrinological, and behavioural illnesses. Many of these have multiple-factor environmental and 'lifestyle' causes and are difficult to assess. With many more women entering the workplace and workers migrating extensively, workforces are becoming much more heterogeneous, thereby complicating risk assessment and management. Reproductive and genetic hazards are very hard to analyze and are especially disturbing.

We need to establish solid health-data baselines upon which to evaluate these concerns. Reproductive issues are a good example: we need to know much more about the incidence of sterility, spontaneous abortion and miscarriage, and premature and low-birthweight birth; about sperm counts, morphology, motility, and enzymology; and about birth defects. In public-health emergencies, such as those at Windscale, Seveso, Love Canal, and Three Mile Island, investigators probe many such indices. We know neither the baseline status for most communities, nor the mechanisms through which harm occurs, nor what would comprise appropriate 'control' populations for comparison. The same analytic limitations afflict chromosome studies, assays of blood 'markers', and psychological evaluation.

Finally, our agenda must prepare us for coming confrontations with the difficult issues of paternalism, self determination, and protective discrimination. 'Discrimination' need not be pejorative. We have always selected people differentially for jobs, military tasks, and other functions. Genetic screening as a condition for employment is raising this social issue, as is debate over how much Clean Air regulation should protect people who suffer from asthma and emphysema. Allergies are common and staggeringly diverse. As we learn more about immunological and other basic characteristics of people, these complexities and diversities will become more evident.

Almost certainly we will want to discriminate between older and younger, the strong-backed and the weak-framed, potential childbearers and those past childbearing, potential fathers and those past fathering, the overweight stroke-prone and the cardiac robust, smokers and non-smokers. This will conflict directly with equal job opportunity and other social goals. We must discuss these issues now, before they grow too far without broad examination and debate.

In accommodating all these changes, lines of assessment and decision-making will have to be redrawn. The partitions between 'safety' bureaus (concerned mainly with acute trauma) and 'industrial hygiene'and medical bureaus in industry and government will have to be lowered. Problems like eyestrain, lower-back pain, and sexual impotence are not so easily compartmentalized. Similarly, hazards such as asbestos and Agent Orange, and illnesses such as spontaneous abortion and chromosomal abberations, are revealing how artificial the division of responsibilities between physicians and public-health authorities is. In many areas this issue is being raised by the shift from heavy manufacturing and service industry: old-fashioned 'safety' departments hardly know how to assess the problems that are turning up now in electronics industries, for instance. Too, corporations that have never thought of themselves as chemical companies are having to adapt to the realization that everything - even small-volume etching compounds, brazing alloys, glues, paints, and dusts - is chemical and must be managed as such.

The overall agenda, as evidenced by our meeting, must cut across hazard categories and across national boundaries. We should not expect to develop a unified, detailed risk policy either within or between countries. But now that people, products, and pollutants are flowing so actively, we must work toward common understanding and, wherever possible, uniform standards. Reduction of acid rain, regulation of pharmaceutical commerce, and maintenance of ocean-dumping regimes need this kind of attention right now.

To conclude, I would once again remind us of the essentially tragic nature of our awarenesses, decisions, and commitments, insisting all the while that we are in many ways better off than ever before, and noting that tragedy *is* humanness.

The difference from the past is that - though it is discomfiting - this conjunction of greatly improved science with heightened societal aspirations now puts us in a position to *manage* aspects of the tragedy as it unfolds. Experts perform centrestage and in the wings. All of us chant from the citizens' chorus.

2
Risks to consumers

LESLEY YEOMANS

Introduction

It may be a platitude to say that we are all consumers, but it is nonetheless true, in the sense that we are all people. As such we face innumerable hazards every day - a hazard being a situation with potential for causing harm. So walking downstairs is a hazard, lifting a heavy saucepan full of boiling water is a hazard, crossing the road is a hazard, even eating and drinking are hazards, since too much of either has potential for causing harm. But we only face a risk if we actually eat or drink too much when there is a probability that we may have indigestion or a hangover - a risk being the probability that a harmful event will occur.

So everyone faces hazards and risks but not everyone is equally equipped to evaluate them, to compare them and put them in perspective. Certain groups are better able to assess risk than others. Among such groups are scientists, industrialists and regulatory authorities. This paper is not about such groups but about average, ordinary people who have some knowledge and understanding of risks but who respond irrationally, out of ignorance and fear and who sometimes behave foolishly, either because they fail to think ahead or because they fall into the trap of saying 'it won't happen to me'. This paper explores both types of response.

How risky is life?

The general atmosphere these days, especially in the press and on television seems to be of unmitigated gloom and disaster, in the sense that people are led to believe that life is highly risky: and what is more that it is more risky than in the past. Scare stories abound - dioxin, DES, asbestos, saccharin, tartrazine, Opren, to name but a few recent examples. Accidents are reported widely and assume more significance than the evidence warrants so that people believe flying is highly risky and that industrial accidents of the Three Mile Island, Seveso or Flixborough type pose a real threat on a large scale for the future. This barrage of information leaves people afraid, bewildered and uncertain. They cannot balance one risk against another, they take no account of the benefits which they receive, nor of the costs involved in setting out to reduce some risks to the absolute minimum.

Life is undoubtedly risky, but is it more so now than in the past? In the most obvious sense it is not. In the developed world people do not 'want' in any really physical sense. They do not need to worry about the basic human needs of food, shelter and clothing. Women do not die in childbirth, infant mortality is low, tuberculosis no longer kills, smallpox has been virtually eradicated. People live longer and, partly because they live longer they die of other things, of heart disease and cancer, which have time to develop in older people. The Third World is catching up with the malnutrition and basic disease. Yet they are faced with enough knowledge about the West to know that some of the technology they are beginning touse, pesticides for example, are regarded with suspicion in the West. So they are tempted to refuse to use them and then face unwelcome consequences.

For example, in the light of the scare stories about DDT, Ceylon banned its use in the 1960s. The country then suffered a severe epidemic of malaria which could have been controlled or even prevented altogether if they had used DDT in an eradication programme. Issues such as this pose problems for both the developed and the Third World but they are not relevant to this discussion of risks to consumers.

Attitudes to risk
Despite man's advanced technology, many people still face real risks from natural disasters - floods, earthquakes, hurricanes, tornadoes. Such risks are not limited to people in the Third World. The consequences of natural disasters can be great - loss of property if not loss life. Yet even today people still seem to have some degree of fatalism in their approach to some risks. They may expect more to be done now than in the past in terms of monitoring so as to give advanced warning of such disasters but they don't blame the event on some responsible authority. It is interesting though that even people who face real risks from natural disasters may still worry about the risk of cancer from food additives.

The overriding fear these days is of cancer. Perceptions about and attitudes to risk are determined by a number of factors identified by Slovic et al. They include whether the risk is controllable or not, whether it is voluntary, the nature of the consequences, whether the risk is immediate or delayed, whether it is observable or not, whether the individual is at risk or society as a whole, whether science can identify the risk or not, whether it is a new or old risk, whether the risk can be reduced.

Seriousness of consequences
People are afraid of cancer because it is a delayed effect and because it is believed to cause death in all circumstances. In other words the outcome is very serious. Thus people do not take the risk of food poisoning so seriously because they think the consequences may be nothing more than an upset stomach for a couple of days. They seem not to appreciate that some people die every year from food poisoning and that if we did not take steps to ensure that *Clostridium botulinium* does not survive processing then many more people would probably die of botulism.

Furthermore, the risk of botulism from cooked meats is seen by food regulatory authorities as being significant enough to warrant the continued use of nitrates and nitrites as preservatives, despite the potential risk of cancer from nitrosamines. But most people see the long term risk of cancer as being greater than the risk of sudden death from botulism. It is no use saying to such people we should be doing more to reduce. They argue that the consequences of food poisoning are slight - an upset stomach for a day or two. They do not see that their loss of earnings could affect their families and they certainly do not see that across a whole country the loss of earnings annually as a result of food poisoning could be very high. This highlights the difference in attitude depending on whether the risk will have consequences for the individual or for society as a whole. The greatest threats are seen as those such as nuclear accidents which could affect both the individual and society and cancer which is perceived as affecting the individual.

Voluntary control

Attitudes also differ depending on whether or not people are in control of the hazard themselves. In the main people are less fearful about hazards which are within their control. Furthermore they seem prepared to take far greater risks when they believe they are in full control.

Sometimes they take foolish and unnecessary risks. For example, transferring anti-freeze from a bulk container to an old lemonade bottle and leaving it on the garage window-sill. People must know it is risky but believe they are in control and therefore the worst will not happen and their child will not be silly enough to drink it. But of course some children do, and die.

There is an apparent inconsistency in attitudes towards whether or not the worst will happen. In the case of risk within their control people assume the worst will not happen; in the case of risks outside their control they assume the worst will happen. So they believe that food additives, pesticide residues, hormones in meat, will give them cancer. Clearly one reason for this inconsistency is the amount of information available to people. Of the order of 6000 people die each year from an accident in the home. The biggest single cause is falls. This is a significant number and is of a totally different order of magnitude compared with the risk of dying from cancer caused by food additives. But people read about cancer and food additives, they read about DES and 2,4,5,-T. They do not read about deaths due to falls in the home.

Regulatory decision-making

People lack sufficient, appropriate information to make comparisons themselves and they lack guidance in making comparisons. They see regulatory authorities in different countries taking different decisions on the basis of the same apparent evidence. So they see the FDA in the States proposing to prohibit saccharin, while the UK and rest of Europe take a definite decision to permit its continued use. The problem is that the nature and amount of information put into the cost-benefit equation varies. Information on toxicology, the economic costs and the benefits are almost certainly put into the equation but there may well be other relevant information which should be considered. Take the case of the use of hormones as growth promotors in meat producing animals. It is arguable that their use is economically important and that the risks will be extremely low if concentrations in meat are very low. This is fine in principle, but what will ensure that concentrations in meat are very low? There is a real risk of misuse and this should be included in the overall equation.

It is a very real risk as has been shown in Europe, where baby foods were found to have DES residues sufficient to cause, in theory, physiological effects in children. DES is banned in Europe and the law was being broken. It probably still is being broken. In other words there is a real risk. People want to see evidence that their interests are first and foremost in the mind of the regulatory authorities, not the interests of big business. People appreciate

hat their demands will have economic consequences for themselves and
society but they say they would be prepared to pay. They have this right.

Absolute safety
They say they would be prepared to pay to make life safer.

Sometimes it seems they are asking for a life to be made absolutely safe.
But this is not so since they want to continue to take the risks they choose to
take. So they want to go on drinking, and smoking, driving, hang-gliding,
motor racing, skiing. But they want things which are outside their control to
be absolutely safe. They may be unrealistic in their attitudes but this is
understandable. They are not even scientists, let alone scientific phil-
osophers, so they have never heard of Karl Popper and do not appreciate
that modern science is based on falsifying theories, not on gathering evidence to prove a theory. They believe that things can be proven to be safe. They
continue to demand this approach furthermore, because they are faced, almost daily,
with evidence that things are not absolutely safe.

The media publishes shock-horror stories about chemicals, drugs, food
additives, asbestos, and people are led to believe that they face a real, daily
threat from such things. It is right that the media should expose the failings
of industry and authority but it is irresponsible to lead the public to imagine
that absolute safety can ever exist. It is particularly irresponsible in the case
of drugs.

The recent Opren story illustrates the point. The message that came
across from the media was that the industry and authorities had failed
because they did not pick up the problems soon enough, nor act on the
evidence when it did come to light. To some extent the criticisms are
probably justified but no one made the crucial point that drugs are biologically active substances and as such are bound to present some risks. It is
a case of balancing one risk against another. Some people suffer a headache
rather than take aspirin, others take aspirin at the first sign of a headache.
There is a danger that some seriously ill people could suffer unnecessarily if
active and effective drugs were withdrawn at the first sign of adverse side
effects.

Science: a dilemma
Scientists must also carry some responsibility for the public's confusion and
uncertainty. On the one hand science is very precise. It can identify with
certainty the most minute amounts of substances. It can find trace amounts
of extremely dangerous substances in almost anything that is examined. On
the other hand, despite this precision, science cannot yet explain the real
significance of such small amounts. Perhaps it really is a case of ignorance
being bliss. In the old days we didn't find dangerous substances so we
assumed they were not there. Or we assumed they were there but didn't
worry because we didn't know for sure. Now we know they are there but
don't know what they mean.

DDT in human breast milk illustrates the problem well. People in West
Germany are particularly concerned about pesticide residues in food. They
have detailed legislation laying down maximum permitted limits for residues in food and so there are limits for DDT residues in meat and milk
products. A few years ago the authorities decided to check on DDT levels in
human breast milk. They found levels which exceeded the maximum permitted limits. But then they didn't know what to do. Maximum permitted

limits are generally regarded as safe limits and so the story was picked up as being unsafe mothers' milk. There was no evidence of this of course. There were no comparative figures over time and the actual amounts were very low. A real dilemma faced the authorities.

The biggest problem for both scientists and authorities is how to interpret the results of toxicity testing and the significance of the presence of minute amounts of substances. They are the experts and people expect them to be certain. It is difficult for the public to accept that experts can be uncertain and fallible. It is difficult to appreciate that precise results do not in themselves provide the answer about what to do next. That is a matter of judgement. It is often the case then that different groups will judge the evidence differently. So the USA proposes a ban on saccharin, while the UK judges its continued use to be acceptable. No one likes having instances where new evidence has resulted in an earlier decision being reversed. The possibility that this may happen in the future is bound to make experts extremely cautious in their approach. They may become unwilling to say 'there is no evidence that this substance poses an undue risk to consumers' and may retreat into asking for more and more evidence. The problem is that they are generally looking at specific, substances within a limited framework - the use of hormones as growth promoters for example, and it is not part of their responsibility to put the question into a larger framework. This should be the responsibility of governments.

Problems for governments
But governments are prone to confusion and uncertainty. They often face conflicting demands from industry and consumers or other special interest groups. Furthermore governments are not independent. They have a political interest to consider, which sometimes overrides other interests.

So governments set up independent expert committees to advise them. But then as often as not choose to ignore the recommendations of the committee. Or they hold public inquiries at which all interests are allowed to state their views but the original decision stands at the end of the day. There is a danger that the independent consultative process will fall into disrepute if decisions seem to be unaffected by views expressed both by the experts and ordinary people. It is equally true that governments have to take some decisions, even in the face of differing views from the majority of people. The most that can be offered is the chance to be heard before the decision is put into effect - consultation.

It is also important that people should have a chance to air their views publicly, not just in private consultation. Emotional, irrational, illogical and inconsistent views may be expressed but at least people have a chance to be heard. There may be reluctance on the part of authorities to hold open, public meetings, because there is a danger that the extreme views of the minority will be picked up by the media and given more attention than they deserve. In giving them such attention other people begin to believe that such views are shared by the majority.

In the field of risk assessment and evaluation the overriding need at present seems to be that of putting all the issues into perspective. Different risks are evaluated by different expert groups and by different parts of government. There is no group to bring them all together. It is by no means sure either that all groups apply the same criteria in their assessment of risk, nor of costs and benefits. It is surely time that a special group was set up to look at all these aspects of risk, and to make recommendations about future policy for risk management.

Conclusions
People face many risks. Some they take in full knowledge of the dangers, others because they think the worst will not happen to them and they believe they face others about which they know nothing.

They are afraid of this last group of risks and cannot put them into perspective alongside the other groups because they lack sufficient knowledge. They face a bewildering array of information about risks but in the main reporting is emotional and prejudiced and does not help people develop a balanced view. Scientists, governments and consumer organisations have a responsibility to help people come to a balanced view about risks but it is not easy to see the best way of achieving this. Public participation in the decision-making process is one way. Decision-making is currently fragmented among different government departments and expert committees.

It is suggested that there is a need for a central policy-making group with the task of reviewing risk generally and of formulating national policies on risk and risk management.

(The views expressed are those of the author and do not necessarily reflect those of the Consumers' Association.)

3
Uncertainties in risk estimation and implications for risk management in industry

R F GRIFFITHS

Introduction

The concept of being at risk is widely understood to mean the condition of being exposed to the chance of an undesirable consequence. This qualitative understanding has existed for a very long time. Alongside this broad understanding quantitative methods have been developed by specialist groups for particular purposes, for example, formulae used by insurance actuaries for the calculation of premiums. Such calculations depend much on the existance of records documenting the occurrence of particular kinds of events, ie quantification requires a large number of case histories. Over the last 10 to 20 years techniques have emerged by means of which it is possible to produce plausible quantitative expressions of risk for classes of events that cannot adequately be assessed on the basis of case histories. This may be because the cause-and-effect chain in individual cases is uncertain (eg carcinogenic effects of chemicals or radioactive materials), or because there have been relatively few actual occurrences (eg major accidents at chemical plants).

Such risks nonetheless give cause for concern, and consideration of the scale and nature of the potential or actual harm associated with them suggests that this concern is reasonable rather than fanciful. Particular events causing varying degrees of harm confirm this view: the Windscale reactor accident of 1957; the Aberfan disaster of 1966; the Flixborough disaster of 1974; the Seveso release of 1976; the Spanish camp-site disaster of 1978; and the accident at the Three-Mile Island reactor in 1979.

The formation of the Advisory Committee on Major Hazards immediately after the Flixborough disaster had a profound effect on this field, and the two reports of 1976 and 1979 have led to the introduction of new regulations (1), effective from 1 January 1983 which partly fulfil the ACMH's recommendations on hazardous installations. Concurrent with these regulatory developments much effort has been evident internationally in the carrying out of generic or site-specific risk assessments for various kinds of installation (eg the USNRC study on nuclear reactors (2); the two reports on Canvey Island (3 and 4); the German study on nuclear reactors (5); the COVO study on chemical plant risks in the Rijnmond area (6)). Major programmes of experimental research have been generated in attempts to improve the basis of technical knowledge used in such studies, for example, numerous field-trials on the release and dispersion of dense gases, sponsored by, amongst others, Shell Research Ltd (7), the Health and Safety Executive (8), and the US Department of Energy (9). Additionally, results of risk assessment studies have been presented as evidence to numerous public enquiries, including the Windscale enquiry of 1977, and the current enquiry on the Sizewell PWR; the Canvey Island risk studies were established as a result of the recommendations of a public enquiry into a planning application to extend oil refining installations at the Canvey site.

Applications that merit a full public enquiry represent only a small fraction of the number of cases involving major hazards that have to be processed each year by the planning departments of Local Authorities. Under a voluntary arrangement first established in the early seventies local planning authorities may now seek advice from the Major Hazards Assessments Unit of the Health and Safety Executive in respect of proposals for new major hazards, or developments in the vicinity of existing major hazards. In 1980 some 3500 cases were referred in this way to the Health and Safety Executive (10). It should be noted that there is no obligation for the Local Authority to refer such cases, nor is the Authority obliged to abide by the advice received from the HSE. This situation has led recently to a most interesting test case (11), which will be discussed further in this paper.

These examples serve to illustrate the scale of the effort and influence associated with this burgeoning field. In view of the nature of the implications for the public, for industry, and for regulatory and technical bodies, it is pertinent to examine some of the uncertainties involved in the assessment of risk in the context of decision-making for major hazards.

Sources of uncertainty
The common feature in the risk quantification studies referred to above is the description of identified risks in terms of two elements, namely the probability of occurrence of the event, and the magnitude or severity of the consequences. The techniques used to produce quantitative expressions of these two aspects can conveniently be divided into (i) methods of analysis of the engineering system itself (drawing on reliability engineering and failure analysis); and (ii) methods for modelling the consequences following release to the environment (particularly dispersion and uptake of hazardous materials).

Details of the methods are reviewed elsewhere (12, 13), or are described in particular studies such as those referred to above. The important feature that makes estimation of uncertainty particularly difficult is that these methods essentially constitute a synthesis of techniques and knowledge drawn from many diverse disciplines, so that a coherent treatment of uncertainty is not available, in the way that it is for, say, the description of errors of observation or variability in a body of physical data. In addition, there are substantial pressures to produce answers of some sort, and where knowledge is uncertain best estimates based on professional or expert judgement are often invoked. Griffiths (14) offers examples of cases where such judgements are called for:

(i) the knowledge of a particular phenomenon which figures in the overall assessment may not yet have been developed beyond the fundamental research stage, in which case reliable predictions of sufficient accuracy may not be possible, eg the atmospheric dispersion of toxic or explosive mixtures that are denser than air.

(ii) the knowledge required is obtainable in principle but it may not be ethically acceptable to undertake the particular investigations that would be required to yield accurate information, eg effects on humans of certain toxic agents.

(iii) uncertainties in the validity of extrapolating from laboratory to industrial-scale systems may have to be accepted because of the economic impractability of undertaking a series of full-scale tests, eg large pressure-vessel failure mechanisms.

In the following sections examples illustrating uncertainties in quantification and assessment will be explored.

Uncertainty in quantification of hazard range
In many studies concerned with major hazards, including most of those cited above, an important aspect of the consequence modelling is the estimation of hazard range for a given release. The principal classes of materials involved are:

(i) radioactive - usually as a mixture of several radionuclides grouped according to physical properties (2);

(ii) combustible materials such as liquified natural gas, or liquified petroleum gas, that may form clouds that will drift considerable distances, constituting a flammable hazard if ignition sources are encoun tered whilst the gas concentration is within the Lower and Upper Flammable Limits (for the LNG the LFL and UFL are 5% and 15% respectively);

(iii) toxic materials such as chlorine, ammonia, phosgene, that are likely to cause injury or death if exposure takes place at concentrations (typically) higher than a few tens or hundreds of parts per million.

In the case of radioactive materials the principal measure of harm is the total dose received, to which either the severity or the probability of occurrence of the harmful effect is related by an appropriate dose-response relationship.

Although there are many complications in such calculations, there seems little doubt that the total dose received from exposure to a radioactive plume dispersing in the atmosphere dominates over secondary factors such as the rate at which that dose is received from the plume. Current models of dispersion used in this context (15) centre on estimates of the time-averaged concentration, and are adequate to the extent that they succeed in predicting that value. A statement of the accuracy of such models requires many qualifications depending on the circumstances of application, but recent comparisons of model predictions and experimental data suggest that even under conditions that do not strain the model, one cannot expect predictions of time-averaged concentration to be much better than within a factor of 2 or 3 of experimental values (16).

In reality, the concentration seen at a point is composed of fluctuations about some average value, often with substantial segments of zero concentration. Such exposures are described as intermittent. Provided the harmful effect can be related satisfactorily to the time-averaged value of concentration, these fluctuations are of little interest in assessing risks. However, consideration of the nature of the hazard posed by combustible materials and by many of the toxic materials of interest in major hazards leads at once to the conclusion that time-averaged estimates of concentration are not sufficient.

For combustible materials the characteristic of crucial importance (given the presence of sources of ignition) is the 'instantaneous' concentration, and its relation to the UFL and the LFL for that particular gas.

The UFL and LFL values for simple mixtures with air are well defined, as for the case of liquified natural gas mentioned above. Clearly it is of little use to know that the time-averaged concentraion takes a particular value at a point unless we know the details of the fluctuating values on which the average is based. This point is well illustrated in experiments carried out by Birch et al (17), reviewed by Chatwin (18), from which Figure 1 is taken. In

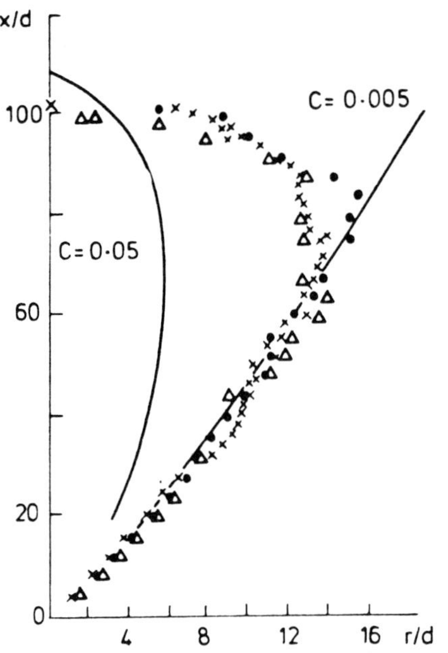

Fig 1. *Flammable boundry for total burn-up of a natural-gas jet (see refs 17 & 18)*

these experiments an ignition source was located at various points in the radial plane of a natural gas jet, and the data points mark the boundary within which the ignition source had to be placed to achieve full burn-up of the jet. The important feature to be noted is that this boundary lies considerably further from the axis than the contour on which the average concentration was 5% (the LFL for the gas).

Further demonstration of this point is obtained from measurements of peak-to-mean ratios of concentration reported by Koopman et al (9), from full-scale experiments involving the release of 40 cubic metre quantities of LNG onto water. Gas concentrations were measured downwind with a time

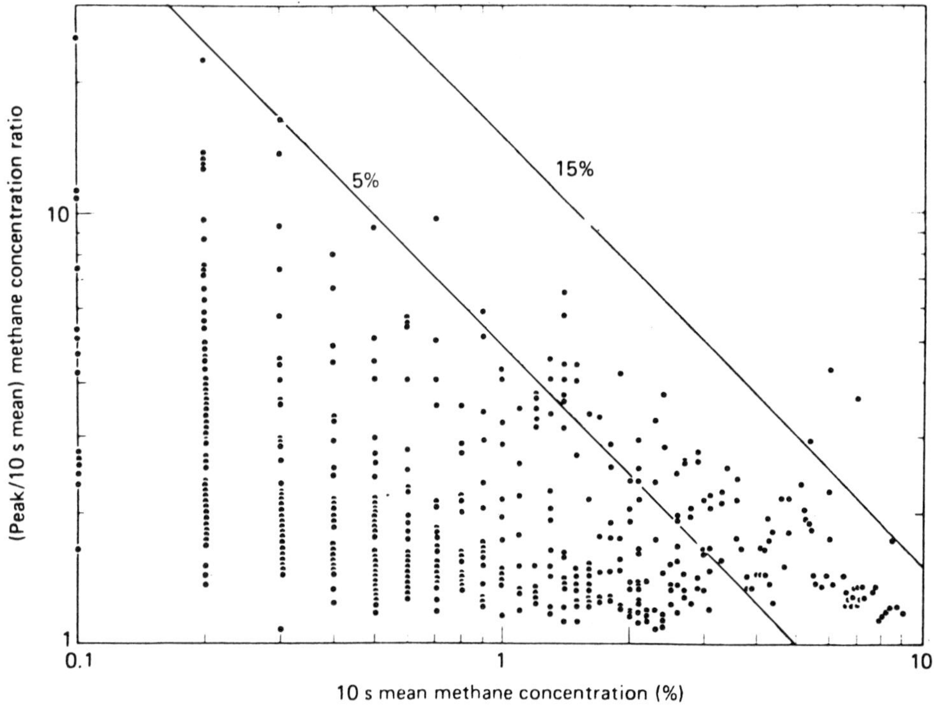

Peak-to-mean concentration ratio vs. mean concentration for Burros 7, 8 and 9.
Points between the diagonal lines are within the flammable limits.

Fig 2. *Peak-to-mean concentration ratios of LNG*
from full-scale test (Koopman et al. ref9)

resolution of 3 to 5 Hz, and from these data 10-second mean values were generated. Figure 2 shows the results of this exercise with peak concentrations falling within the flammable range of values ofthe 10-second mean down to 0.3%. In presenting such results it is, of course, very important to specify the averaging time, and the response time of the peak measurements. The trend in Figure 2 for the peak-to-mean ratio to increase as the mean decreases should be noted. Jones (19) has recently examined the effect of response time by applying various low-pass filters to a set of concentration data taken with a very fast (0.1 kilohertz) response detector.

Although strictly applicable only to the very short downwind ranges used in his experiments, the results show concentration ratios ranging from 2 to 20 at the 95% cumulative probability level as the response times. These considerations strongly suggest that to define the maximum hazard range in terms of a time-averaged estimate of the LFL contour will result in an underestimate of the true extent of the flammable cloud. The dispersion models currently in use for such estimates (see reviews by Blackmore et al (20) and Woodward et al (21)) make no attempt to describe dispersion in terms of concentration fluctuations. Whilst it is probably premature (in terms of required knowledge) to develop such improved models, it is important to be aware of the likely limitations of present techniques, especially since they probably lead to over-optimistic estimates.

In the case of toxic materials, such as some of the irritant gases of importance in major hazards, the situation is complicated yet further by the fact that one cannot readily specify a measure that marks a boundary between 'harmful' and 'not harmful', ie there is no simple equivalent to the UFL and LFL values for combustibles. For many toxic gases the appropriate expression of toxic response is in the form of a relationship between the concentration, C, and duration of exposure, T, and the percentage of the exposed population that might suffer a particular level of damage. This is known as the probit function, which takes the form

$$P = a + b \ln (Cnt)$$

The quantity P is related to the percentage of the exposed population that suffer a given effect. This method of describing susceptibility to toxic substances was originally developed to express results of experiments on the effectiveness of insecticides, and is the subject of an authoritative text by Finney (22). In principle one can specify various levels of harm ranging

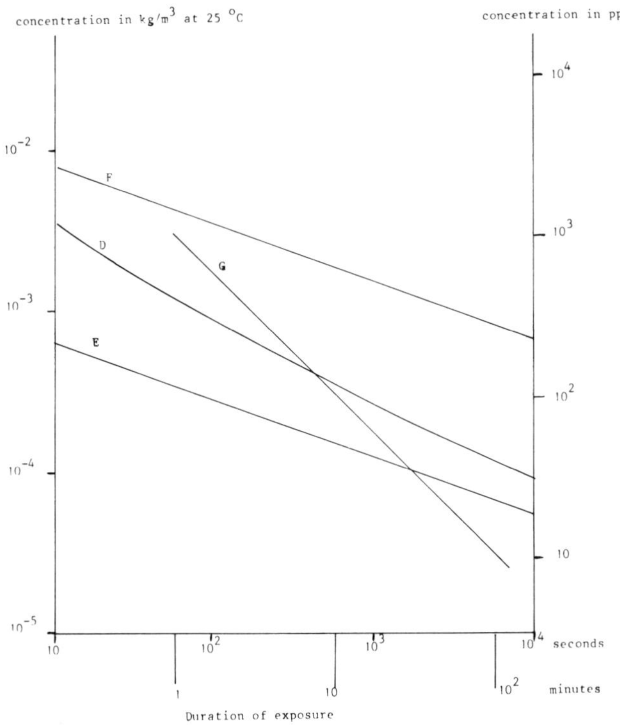

Fig 3. *LD 50 values for chlorine, from various sources:*

D) Dicken, A.N.A. The quantitative assessment of chlorine emission hazards, Chlorine Bicentennial Symposium, San Francisco, Chlorine Institute, 244-256, 1974. E) Eisenburg, N.A. et al Vulnerability model, a simulation system for assessing damage resulting from marine spills, NTIS report AD-A015-245, 1975. F) COVO report (reference 6 in main list) section 5-28. G) Chlorine Institute personal communication given in Simmons, J.A., Erdmann, R.C. and Naft, B.N., Risk assessment of large spills of toxic materials Conf. on control of hazardous material spills, San Francisco, 166-175, 1974.

22

from, say, mild irritation through reversible damage to fatal; for each specified effect there will be a set of values for the coefficients a and b, and the
index n. Proper use of the probit method requires comprehensive data on
exposure and response, obtainable from many applications by direct experiment.

However, it will cause no surprise to note that the data available for
human toxic response are extremely sparse. Nontheless, several reviews
have been carried out in attempts to interpret these data and values of the
necessary quantities have been proposed in the literature, and used in
various risk studies. We have recently conducted an examination of these
studies and have found wide variations in the toxicity models used for
ammonia, and for chlorine. Full details will be reported in a paper currently
under preparation (23), but an illustrative example will demonstrate the
conclusion that this source of uncertainty is substantial. Figure 3 is a compilation of LD50 values for exposure to chlorine. These combinations of
concentration and duration of exposure were fed into a computer model of
dispersion suitable for dense gas mixtures (DENZ, described in reference
24). The output of the programme specifies hazard ranges and areas within
which the specified level is exceeded. Figure 4 shows the results obtained

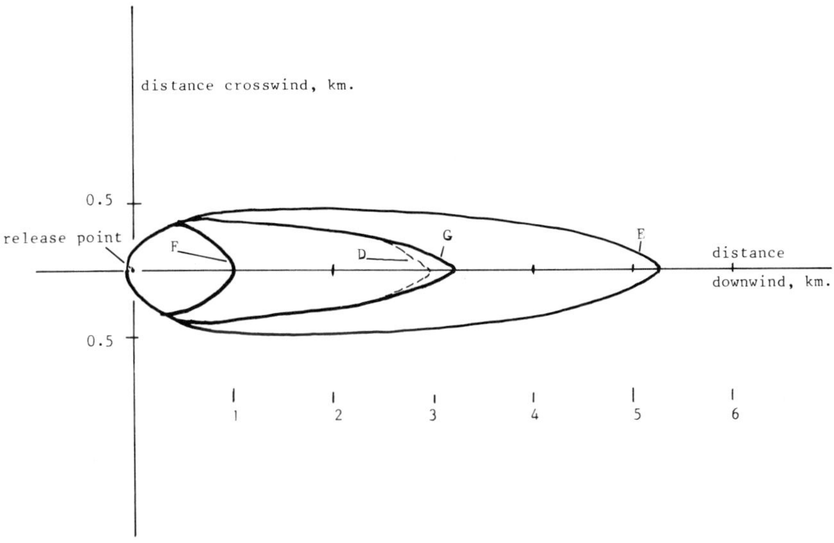

Fig 4. LD 50   *Contours calculated using the four toxic response models illustrated in Figure 3 for a 50 tonne release
of chlorine under class D met conditions with a windspeed of m/sec*

using the four LD50 graphs displayed in Figure 3 for a notional sudden
release of 50 tonnes of chlorine in class D meteorological conditions (with
windspeed 5 m/sec). Class D is the most prevalent weather condition in the
UK. The downwind range to the LD50 is seen to vary between 1.0 and 5.3 km,
a factor of approximately 5 between extreme values. Under other meteorological conditions the range of predictions for the LD50 differed by factors

as high as 10. It is clear from these results that lack of reliable knowledge on the toxicity of materials such as chlorine is a crucial factor in the uncertainty of hazard range prediction. It should be emphasised that other levels, such as the LD05 and the LD95, are subject to similar factors of uncertainty, and there is no particular reason to choose the LD50 as the reference level.

The discussion above emphasises the range of uncertainty associated with particular ways of specifying what is meant by hazard range. The reference point to which these uncertainties apply is, in most studies, the particular concentration contour predicted by a dispersion model. The models used in this field produce a single answer given a specified set of input data, and do not allow for the fact that dispersion is a statistical process that may in practice yield a range of results under nominally identical conditions. Several attempts have been made to compare model predictions with the results obtained in full-scale field trials, with a view to testing the validity of the model (21). Although it is the case that some models yield results that compare well with particular experiments, it should be noted that one is usually limited to the results of a single experiment with which to make comparisons.

This is a consequence of the practical difficulties involved in such field experiments, in which it is rarely possible to run tests under the precise meteorological conditions that may have been prescribed in the experimental design, and, therefore, repetitions of a particular experiment are almost unattainable in practice. A significant insight into this problem is available from results of wind tunnel simulations (25) of the Porton dense gas trials (26). In the wind tunnel tests it was possible to repeat particular runs under nominally identical conditions. In one experiment 20 repeats were carried out, and the results showed a factor of 9 variation in the maximum concentration measured at a point over the 20 runs. This result suggests that the apparent validity claimed for some models on the basis of comparisons with single tests is likely to require much more stringent demonstration before it can be accepted as a basis for risk quantification.

Discussion
The above considerations deal only with one factor (ie consequence modelling) necessary in risk quantification, and say nothing about the uncertainties associated with estimating the probability of the release occurring in the first place. This is not to dismiss the importance of this source of uncertainty, which could be expected to lead to factors of similar magnitude. However, the arguments presented here are sufficient to raise doubts as to the validity of estimates of hazard range quoted to the nearest metre, as in the recent COVO report (6). It is relatively easy to find examples suggesting that the methodology of risk assessment has taken over from the user, bringing to mind the observation usually attributed to Gauss, that the lack of mathematical culture is revealed nowhere so conspicuously as in meaningless precision in numerical computations. A less delicate expression of the same sentiment is to be found in the industrial comments section of the COVO report (6, p 692): 'Whether it is cost effective to spend enormous amounts of money in calculating useless data is not for us to judge'.

Whilst such sweeping statements may not be fully justified, it is easy to sympathise with the sense of exasperation that is expressed. The response of industry to this situation has been very mixed; some organisations have contributed very substantial resources to improve our knowledge of technical aspects involving risk, whilst others have chosen simply to reserve their position.

This brings us to consider the complicated relationship between the public, industry and the authorities of local and central government. It is often said that the public perception of risk is distorted compared with 'real' risk. What is meant by real risk? Some industrialists argue that the historical record of accidents is what counts, and that risk analysis gives pessimistic results. Risk analysts respond that the models used are reasonable and that for events of low probability the historical record does not give a full picture of the risk potential. Both views represent valid contributions to the debate. The danger is when any party takes an entrenched position in either extreme, seeking illusory justification either in the sanctity of overworked analytical models, or in the incomplete picture of the statistical record. The inquiry referred to earlier of the same sentiment is to be found in the industrial comments (11), provides an object lesson in this field.

A developer proposed to build a housing estate close to a plant where chlorine and phosgene were used. The local authority received advice from the Health and Safety Executive, but chose to ignore that advice and grant permission. The Health and Safety Executive pressed the issue and a public enquiry was opened. The inspector recommended in favour of the applicant, and criticised the Health and Safety Executive in his report. The Secretary of State accepted the inspector's advice and permission was granted. In view of the uncertainties involved in hazard prediction one can sympathise with the Health and Safety Executive's difficult position, obliged to give advice, but clearly not wishing to put its faith in numbers. One can equally well understand the position adopted by the industrial body involved, which was to emphasise the facts of the safety record. All this leaves the local authorities in a most difficult position; as expressed by Brough (27), 'Central government advice is not adequate for my council's purposes'.

Some progress has been made in researching technical topics, and in publishing risk assessment reports. However, such exercises are expensive. The first Canvey study cost about £400 000, and the COVO study was about the same. The Rasmussen report cost £4 million. Field experiments on dense gas dispersion cost typically £1 million for a half-dozen full-scale releases, and massive man-year expenditure goes into the planning application procedures.

It would be very satisfying to be able to offer a tidy solution to this complex problem, but that solution is not at hand. What is clear, though, is that the uncertainty associated with the technical aspects is greater than one would conclude from some of these studies recently published.

While this uncertainty remains it is inappropriate to consider risks in rigid terms. A comprehensive view is needed, and those involved may need more time to examine the wider view. This will not make their task easier, but it will make for a more balanced basis for decision, and hopefully it will lead to a greater understanding of what risk assessment can and cannot do.

References

1. The notification of installations handling hazardous substances regulations 1982, Statutory Instrument No 1357, 1982.
2. USNRC, Reactor Safety Study (The Rasmussen Report), USNRC, Washington DC, 1975.
3. HSE, Canvey - and investigation of potential hazards from operations in the Canvey Island-Thurrock area, HMSO, London,1978.
4. HSE, Canvey - a second report, HMSO, 1981.
5. The German Risk Study, Gesellschaft für Reaktorsicherheit, Garching, 1979.
6. COVO report, Risk Analysis of six potentially hazardous industrial objects in the Rijnmond area, Reidel, 1982.
7. Puttock, J S et al. Field experiments on dense gas dispersion. J Haz Mat, 6,13-41,1982.
8. McQuaid, J. Future directions of dense gas dispersion research. J Haz Mat, 6, 231-247, 1982.
9. Koopman, R P et al. Analysis of Burro series 40 m3 LNG spill experiments. J Haz Mat, 6, 43-83, 1982.
10. Pantony M F and Smith, L M. An example of HSE's assessment of major hazards as an aid to planning control by local authorities. I Chem E Symposium Series No 71, 377-395, 1982.
11. Inspector's Report. Application by Broseley Estates Ltd (Wyre Borough Council) Depts of the Environment and Transport, 1982.
12. McCormick N J. Reliability and risk analysis. Academic Press, 1981.
13. Lees, F P. Loss prevention in the process industries. Butterworths, 1980.
14. Griffiths, R P. (ed) Dealing with risk. Manchester University Press, 1981.
15. NRPB. A model for short and medium range dispersion of radionuclides released to the atmosphere. NRPB Report R91, 1979.
16. Barker, C D. A comparison of the Gaussian plume diffusion model with experimental data from Tilbury and Northfleet. CEGB Report RD/B/N4624, 1979.
17. Birch, A D et al. Ingition probabilities in turbulent mixing flows. British Gas Report No MRS E 374, 1980.
18. Chatwin, P C. The use of statistics in describing and predicting the effects of dispersing gas clouds. J Haz Mat, 6, 213-230, 1982.
19. Jones, C D. On the structure of instantaneous plumes in the atmosphere. J Haz Mat, 7,87-112, 1983.
20. Blackmore, D R, Heavy gas dispersion models. J Haz Mat, 6, 107-128, 1982.
21. Woodward, J L. A comparison with experimental data of several models for dispersion of heavy vapour clouds. J Haz Mat, 6, 161-180, 1982.
22. Finney, D J. Probit analysis. Cambridge University Press, 1952.
23. Griffiths R P and Megson, L C. Paper under preparation.
24. Fryer, L S and Kaiser, G D. DENZ - a computer program for the calculation of the dispersion of dense toxic or explosive gases in the atmosphere. UKAEA Report SRD R152, 1979.
25. Hall, D J et al. A wind tunnel model of the Porton dense gas spill field trials. Warren Spring Laboratory Report LR 394 (AP), 1982.
26. Picknett, R G. Dispersion of dense gas puffs released in the atmosphere at ground level. Atm Env 15, 509-525, 1981.
27. Brough, C W. Dealing with hazard and risk in planning. In Griffiths, R F. (ed) Dealing with risk. Manchester University Press, 1981.

Note
References 7,8,9,18,20 and 21 are also published in a compilation of papers under the title 'Dense gas dispersion', Britter R E and Griffiths, R F. (eds) Chem Eng Monographs No 16, Elsevier Scientific Publishing Company, Amsterdam, 1982.

4
Risk, age and society

PETER H MILLARD

The desire to avoid regret later governs our actions. In taking risks the person who gambles has to be able to live with himself afterwards and in trying to avoid risk he sometimes hides within the anonymity of the group.

I am honoured to have been invited to address such a distinguished audience on the subject of risk, age and society, but am all too conscious of the risk that I am taking. I have crashed once before - will it occur again? Will I reach the expectation of the organisers and of you, the audience? Such fears race through one's mind and sometimes they can be so strong that they paralyse all action.

I have to accept some responsibility for my actions, although the decision to ask me to speak was that of the organising body, but I accepted, I can no longer hide - I must stand and talk.

Cicero, writing about public speaking states: 'The better qualified a man is to speak, the more he fears the difficulty of speaking, the uncertain success of his speech, and the expectation of the audience'.

My qualifications to speak on risk, ageing and society arise from my professional employment as a doctor with special responsibility for the aged and I am all too conscious of my lack of qualifications.

In writing this paper, I have drawn upon the experience gained in taking risks with aged people. The word 'risk' found its way into the English language in the 17th century and is thought to have been originally a sailor's term - from the Spanish - 'to run into danger' or 'go against a rock'.

That the origins are nautical is not surprising because the first example of the risk business was the money used to fund shipments overseas - in the early days of travel, a risky business.

The word risk is now used to imply a hazard, a chance of loss expecially the loss of property or goods in insurance. Some risks can be mathematically calculated. Others cannot. The word 'hazard', for example, comes from the Arabic and means to gamble with dice - because dice are six-sided - the chances of losing can be worked out. The bookmaker always wins, but the man who gambles his money is dominated by hopes of success coupled with fears of losing. He feels regret if he does not bet and he discovers later that he would have won, and remorse if he did bet and lost.

Life is a risky business. If only we had done something - we could have stopped the child from drowning - can soon become legislation that 'children may not go near water'. Or if we had not discharged the old lady she would not have fallen down and broken her leg becomes 'all patients must stay in hospital'. Then of course nobody goes home and nobody can come in - but that is not our fault for the Government should have provided more beds. The specialty of geriatric medicine exists because in 1948 Government legislated that the sick, aged patients who needed nursing care were the responsibility of the NHS. The reason for this was the evidence that the chronic sick were misdiagnosed and mismanaged in local authority-run long-stay wards. Until 1948 the medical management of these patients was the responsibility of the general practitioner but now it is a specialist task. Arising fron the decision to allocate responsibility, the whole new specialty of Geriatric Medicine exists.

In just over thirty years, the achievements have been staggering. Wards have been transformed from warehouses where the unwanted bodies of the aged were tended in bed - to hives of activity where doctors, nurses, therapists and porters work together in teams to help the aged patient to regain their physical mobility and thus become less dependent.

At first one patient used to occupy a bed for the whole year, now five are treated. Departments have been reorganised. Home visiting by hospital staff, Day Hospitals and after-discharge teams have been developed.

This was not achieved without taking risks or without making mistakes. One major mistake was the excessive use of cot-sides to prevent people falling out of high beds and thus it was that patients fell from an even greater height to the floor. The proper solution was adjustable height beds!

Encouraging elderly people to become independent means that risks have to be taken which could result in their falling and breaking a leg. The child has the ability to right itself rapidly when it stumbles and even if it does fall the bones are springy and rarely broken. In the aged however the ability to right oneself rapidly on falling is lost, each stumble can mean a fall and aged bones are rigid and easily broken.

Rigidity is a characteristic of age. Age may bring with it wisdom, acquired through knowledge. But does the wisdom one has acquired through making mistakes eventually paralyse the old and the young? In my family one dominant fear is motorbikes. My mother had it, I have it, my children have it. The special distinction of civilised man is foresight and co-operation. To be forewarned is to be forearmed. Thus man is able to make himself safe from others. For the savage, life is a lottery - if one has to hunt for food all one's interests are at risk - but as civilisation progresses the element of chance is slowly eliminated from life. In a progressive society, education, science, invention, regular government and civil order steadily work together to narrow the realm of chance and extend that of foresight. Nothing happens, because no risks are taken. The all seeing, all powerful, all embracing state takes over, the risks are eliminated, no more chances are taken and the society dies.

The fruit fly lives and dies in 75 days, the mouse in 400 days, the dog in twelve years, the human in a hundred years and civilisations in 700 to a thousand years.

The proper study of mankind is man. What is so surprising about our society is that we legislate for the present but do not learn from the past. Ancient Egyptian, Greek and Roman civilisations all went through periods of birth, growth, maturity, decay and death. A characteristic of their decline and fall was legislative rigidity.

Everthing ages - nothing escapes. Plants and animals, machines and men, families, societies and nations all age. Consider for a moment an old car - age has effected all its systems; its design is outmoded, body work dented and rusty, interior shabby, some instruments don't work, and multi-system failure is frequent in its mechanical parts. Unwanted it lies on the scrapheap and yet once it was a man's pride and joy. For some it had been the very symbol of their status - rather than just a means of transport. In the hands of an enthusiast it can be transformed into something to be admired but most of us do not care and it dies. Death is the end of our mortal existence and thus it is that society wages an unending warfare against premature death from any cause.

Must societies inevitably die - must rigidity and death go hand in hand with ageing?

The disengagement theory of ageing which arises from a study of business life states that a man sets off in his life hoping to change the world in his lifetime, then realising he cannot he becomes a raconteur prior to surrounding himself with rigid rules prior to retirement from work.

Is the increasing protective legislation a sign of an ageing society? More and more legislation tries to eliminate risk and the structure of society gradually becomes more rigid. Now trade unions defend their members rights, outmoded machines are preserved, and the specialist societies surround themselves with more and more examinations.

Perhaps the hazard warning for all of us should not be related to toxic chemicals but one that states 'beware hazard ahead. Your society is in danger'.

Organisations and societies become rigid with age to protect themselves and to defend their position and status. In that they are no different to humans.

Abraham Maslow, an American psychologist, ranked human needs into five major groups; physiological, safety, love and belonging, esteem and self-fulfilment. He hypothesised that one had to fulfil 90% of each need before one could worry about the next.

The basic need of man is physiological: the need for food and water. Primitive man cannot obtain this without hunting and it is not until agriculture is developed that one can stay at home and worry about one's need for safety.

This established, one needs to be loved and to belong to a group. Group identity, the family, the tribe, the church, the town, the country. Then one aspires to be looked up to, to be respected and held in esteem by others. Finally at the end of one's life one needs to look back on a job well done and have a sense of personal achievement and fulfilment.

We must, however, remember that although we are dead the society lives on and in eliminating risk and consolidating our own achievements we run the risk of destroying society.

5

Now or later? A numerical comparison of short and long-term hazards

TREVOR KLETZ

Introduction

In the Loss Prevention Symposium held in Newcastle in 1971, I presented one of the first papers (1) on the use of numerical methods for comparing the different risks to which employees in the process industries are exposed. Since then such methods have been used for setting priorities between different acute risks and the literature on the subject is now extensive (2-10). In this paper I suggest an extension of these methods to hazards which take a long time, typically several decades, to produce their effects.

Consider a substance X, the product of an industrial process, which can cause harm in two distinct ways:

(A) It may leak out of the plant, vaporise, mix with air and be ignited, thus injuring or killing people by fire or explosion. Very small leaks do not matter: the hazard arises only if the leak exceeds several kg and is unlikey to be serious unless it exceeds 1 tonne (though smaller leaks can be serious in confined spaces).

B) Exposure of employees to small quantities of the vapour for long periods for many years may cause industrial disease which may lead to premature death. In general, we are not concerned with the occasional large release but with the small quantities present in the atmosphere as the result of minute leaks from joints, glands, sample and drain points, maintenance operations and so on. (However, for some materials occasional large doses may produce long-term effect, or may cause sensitisation.)

The Threshold Limit Value (TLV) gives the time-weighted average concentration for a normal 8-hour work-day or 40-hour work-week, to which nearly all workers may be repeatedly exposed, day after day, without adverse effect. It does not, of course, provide a sharp division between safe and unsafe conditions.

We try, of course, to prevent both sorts of leak and we spend a lot of money and effort in doing so. How does our success in overcoming hazard (A) compare with our success in overcoming hazard (B)? We do not know.

Should we put more effort into preventing the occasional big leaks or more effort into preventing the continuous small leaks? We do not know. Usually different people, using different criteria and financed by different budgets, are responsible for dealing with the two hazards. Finding a way of talking to them both at the same time is like finding a way of communicating, at the same time, to people who speak different languages. This is attempted in this paper.

The problem is not just one of comparing risks. It is made more difficult by the fact that the risks are different and are felt to be different by those who are subjected to them. Suppose that the probabilities of an employee being killed by the acute hazard (A) and the chronic or long-term hazard (B) are equal. An employee might feel that hazard (B) leaves him with an extra 20 or more years of life and therefore further resources should be spent on reducing the risk from hazard(A). On the other hand another employee might feel that a fire or explosion is soon over while industrial disease may mean years of worry, wondering whether or not he will contract it, possibly followed by many years of illness and reduced quality of life.

From society's point of view, long-term hazards, though they may kill many people will kill them over a long period of time and will not produce the same trauma or public outcry as one that kills many people at a time.

In one important respect, the problem of long-term effects differs from all other industrial problems - often the size of the problem is not known. As we shall see in Section 5, we do not know how many people die or suffer from industrial disease (of all sorts, not just the legally prescribed diseases), because the same diseases usually also have non-occupational causes. Before we spend resources on, say, reducing the usage of raw materials or energy, improving product quality, or preventing accidents, we start by asking ourselves what is the present usage, quality, accident rate, etc and what is the scope for improvement. When dealing with toxicological hazards we do not seem able to do this.

A personal note
I have some experience of industrial accidents but little knowledge of toxicology. In trying to compare the two I may be accused, like everyone else who tries to compare two subjects normally considered apart, of dabbling in a field in which I am no expert. I admit the accusation, but if we want to knock a hole in a wall, we have to start from one side.

Some may argue that immediate deaths and delayed deaths are so different that they cannot be compared. However, *comparing different things is what management is about.*

Managers have to set priorities between different sorts of tasks. The question is not whether we compare short and long-term hazards but whether we do so openly and explicitly or inwardly, using unknown criteria (unknown to ourselves as well as to others).

Let us look at some examples, starting with those where the size of the problem is known.

1. Coal dust

This substance is not of great interest to the process indusries but it is the cause of serious industrial disease - in 1975 out of 802 deaths from prescribed industrial disease in the UK, 643 were due to pneumoconiosis, most of it caused by coal dust - and it is one of the few substances for which the dose-response relationship is known. The National Coal Board have shown (11) that:

$$P = \sin^2 (0.0704 \, x - 0.1201)$$

where x = mean respirable dust concentration in mg/m^3

P = probability of developing category 2/1
pneumoconiosis (ILO classification)
in 35 years

When calculating the sine, the expression in the brackets is assumed to beradians.

The equation is based on a statistical extrapolation of observations over ten years in twenty coal mines and mean coalface dust concentrations in those mines up to 8 mg/m^3

In 1970 the National Coal Board set standards which implied that long-term concentrations experienced by individuals would not exceed 4.3 mg/m^3 The corresponding value of P is 9.42 x 10^{-4} per person per year. This would be equivalent to a fatal accident rate (FAR) of 50 or 100 deaths per 10^5 per year, if we asume that all cases of category 2/1 pneumoconiosis lead to premature death.

However, by no means all cases of category 2/1 pneumoconiosis lead to premature death. According to the Institute of Occupational Medicine (12), over 22 years men in the 25-34 year age group with categories 1, 2 and 3 pneumoconiosis had survival rates of 90.1 percent compared with 93 percent for those with category 0. The difference, they state, is statistically significant and suggests that the mortality risk for those with simple pneumoconiosis is about 60 percent higher than that experienced by young men with no radiological signs initially.

What happens after 22 years is not known. Let us therefore assume that ultimately one in three of those with simple pneumoconiosis dies prematurely (though the time of death may be many years ahead).

The pneumoconiosis death rate is then equivalent to a FAR of 17 or 33 deaths per 10^5 men per year.

For comparison the FAR for all acute accidents in coal mines was 40 (80 deaths per 10^5 men per year) in the 1960s but fell to about 14 (28 deaths per 10^5 men per year) in the 1970s.

A coal miner joining the industry is thus about as likely to die from pneumoconiosis than from an acute accident, if past trends continue.

This suggests that the Coal Board has got the allocation of priorities between short and long-term hazards about right.

However, for a man aged 20-24 the total probability of death from all causes (including natural causes) is 10^{-3}/year (13). If he is a coal miner acute industrial accidents increase this by a factor of three. Pneumoconiosis also increases his risk of death by a factor of three but this will probably not take effect for about 40 years by which time his total probability of death from all causes has risen by 20 times to 20 x 10^{-3}/year. Looked at this way the risk of death from pneumoconiosis does not seem as bad as the risk of death from acute industrial accidents.

On the other hand, it could be argued that our hypothetical coal miner may have looked forward to his retirement for 40 years and that death at the time of his retirement is worse than an early death.

This example shows that we cannot assume that probability of death is necessarily the right parameter for use in comparing immediate and delayed effects. Many people may consider that delayed death is preferable; others may take the opposite view. The National Coal Board's actions imply that an immediate death is equivalent to a delayed death. Whatever our views, they seem to have got the balance between acute and chronic risks right to well within an order of magnitude. (Incidentally, halving the coal dust concentration will decrease the incidence of 2/1 pneumoconiosis by about 20 times.)

2.Radiation

This is another area where good dose-response data are available though there is some doubt as to whether it can be extrapolated to low concentrations. For employees the agreed maximum dose is 50 mSv/y (5 rem/y) which is believed to give a risk of death of 5x 10-4/y (FAR 25 or 50 deaths per 10^5 men/y). This seems high compared with acute risks particuarly as people exposed to radioactivity are presumably also exposed to normal acute industrial risks as well. If we assume that the FAR for these acute risks is 2 (as in the chemical industry and most UK manufacturing industries) then those who set nuclear standards are implying that an immediate death is about twelve time worse than a delayed death. Kinchin (15) a former head of the Safety and Reliability Directorate of the UK Atomic Energy Authority, has suggested levels of risk which are so low that action to reduce them further is not justified; his figure for delayed deaths is 30 times higher than his figure for immediate deaths.

Reissland and Harries (16) have suggested, when taking radiation as an example, that loss of expectation of life should be used for comparing risks instead of the probability of deaths. The Table, based on their data, shows that for a man aged 35 or more exposed to 50 mSV/y the acute risks are worse than the chronic risks (assuming as before that he is exposed to the same acute risks as in the other industries).

Table . *Loss of expectation of life for various risks*

Risk *	FAFR	Deaths/10^5 men/year	Loss of expectation of life (days) Age at beginning of exposure (yrs)				
			20	30	40	50	60
Acute							
UK Manuf. Industry	2	4	20	3.5	8	4	1
Chemical Industry * *	4	8	41	27	16	8	2
Chronic							
Exposure to 50 mSv radiation per year	25	50	68	32	12	3	0.5

***Assuming exposure continues for rest of working life**

****and all premises covered by Factories Act**

However, as Griffiths (17) points out, loss of life expectancy is misleading. Consider a group of 1000 men. All of them could lose 10 days life or one man could lose 10 000 days (27 years) but the average loss of life-expectancy is the same. In no way can the two cases be considered similar. To quote Harold Wilson 'For the man who is unemployed, the unemployment rate is 100 per cent.'

3. Asbestos

The UK Threshold Limit Value of 2 fibres per ml for white asbestos was set following a study (18) which showed that one percent of those exposed to this concentration for a working lifetime will develop asbestosis. If we assume that every case of asbestosis results in premature death, this is equivalent to a FAR of 10 (20 deaths per 10^5 men per year). This seems high compared with the acute risks to which asbestos workers are also exposed but actual doses are probably a good deal lower than threshold limit values and by no means all cases of asbestosis result in premature death. Unfortunately very little data are available on the ratio between actual and permitted exposures. (Coal dust is an exception, according to Reference 11 the ratio of average to peak exposure is about 1-2.)

If we assume that the average exposure is one-fifth of the TLV, that is, 0.4 fibre/ml and if we also assume that the dose-response relationship is linear, then 0.2 percent of those exposed will develop asbestosis. This is equivalent to an FAR of 2 if all cases result in premature death (which they do not). (The figure of one-fifth is just an example; I do not know the true figure which will differ from one factory to another.)

It must be remembered that asbestos can cause other diseases besides asbestosis but dose-response data are not available.

4. Chemicals

For chemicals very little accurate dose-response data are available. Roach (19) points out that there are 612 substances in the 1976 ACGIH list of TLVs. Of these, 63 TLVs are based on industrial surveys, of which only 8 involve more than 200 people, and 50 are based on laboratory studies on volunteers.

This sparsity of data is often quoted as a reason for not using hazard analysis (see, for example, Reference 20). However, TLVs are set despite the lack of data, and if there is enough information to set a TLV it should be possible to estimate a probability of death. The probability may err on the safe side, but even so, we can still compare this probability with that of acute accidents. (Some TLVs are based on the concentration required to risk irritation, not risk to life. These are not the ones with which I am concerned. When a TLV is based on a risk to life, if it is possible to set a TLV it should be possible to estimate the risk to life.)

In applying hazard analysis to acute problems it is also often necessary to use expert judgement to fill gaps in the data. If we break problems down into component questions (What was the dose of A? For how long did it continue? What is the effect of such a dose?), answering them with facts where possible and with expert opinion when no facts are available, we are more likely to get a correct answer than if we try to answer the whole problem by expert opinion. Such opinions should be used as substitutes for unavailable data rather than as an alternative method of problem solving.

An attempt to compare acute and long-term risk has been made for workers exposed to benzene (Mountfield, 21). He shows that exposure to 10-1000 ppm produces FARs of 1-10(2-20 deaths per 10^5 men per year), but that there is no evidence that exposure below 10 ppm produces any excess risk. This is confirmed by a recent extensive review by Fielder (22).

This brings us to the question of linearity on which expert opinion is divided (23). Some writers believe that the effect of a toxic chemical is proportional to the dose and that even one molecule (or one photon of radiation) can cause disease, though the probability is small (24). Others consider that there is a threshold dose below which there is no effect, the body's natural defence mechanism coping with the alien material; only when the body's defence mechanism is overwhelmed does disease result. It may be that the response is linear for some substances or effects (for example carcinogens) but that there is a threshold for others (for example coal dust).

The argument cannot be settled epidemiologically as at low doses the effects are too small to be detectable above the background noise, that is, the naturally occurring incidence of the disease. In most cases a TLV may be exceeded but only for a short time. A man should not be exposed to twice the TLV for 4 hours and then to a nil concentration for another 4 hours. This implies that the dose-response data may not be linear at these concentrations, and that low doses produce less effect than would be expected by extrapolation from high doses.

However, in making comparisons of the type discussed in this paper it would be prudent at the present time to base them on a linear hypothesis.

5. All industry

Can we derive any useful information by looking at UK industry as a whole? For 1975-78 the average number of deaths from industrial accidents was 694/y and the average number of deaths from prescribed industrial disease was 925/y (1974-78) (25). This suggests that over industry as a whole, accidents and disease are problems of comparable magnitude. However, about 800 deaths/y out of the 925 are due to pneumoconiosis, asbestosis and byssinosis, diseases restricted to a few industries and occupations. This suggests that acute accidents are the manor problem.

However, the figures for industrial disease include only those due to prescribed disease (26.) Some deaths will be due to non-prescribed diseases but there is no consensus of opinion on the number. Considering cancer alone, one report (27) estimated that one percent of male deaths from cancer (that is, 0.3 percent of all male deaths or 1000 per year) might have occupational causes. Other reports (28-30) have suggested much larger figures. Thus Reference 29 states that 5 percent of all male deaths in the US are due to occupational cancers while Reference 26 suggests 3-6 percent (10 000-20 000 per year) for the UK. These latter reports have been extensively criticised (31) ('It (Reference 29) shows how a group of reasonable men can collectively generate an unreasonable report'), and the Royal Society report seems more likely to be correct.

The 1000 male deaths from occupational cancer per year will include some of those due to prescribed disease; there will be some deaths due to non-prescribed diseases besides cancer, hence it seems that the total number of deaths per year due to occupational disease is perhaps between 1000 and 2000. The uncertainty in the data is illustrated by the fact that the TUC state 'Every year about 1400 people die as a result of occupational accidents and diseases' (32), while Farmer writes 'On a conservative estimate (cancer) kills twice as many work people as industrial accidents' (33). Death from occupational disease is thus a problem comparable with, perhaps rather worse than, death from industrial accidents and justifies appropriate allocation of resources.

Note that deaths from industrial disease reflect the working conditions of many years ago.

If we compare days lost due to industrial accidents with days lost due to industrial disease, we find that in 1976/77 accidents caused 12.2×10^6 lost days while prescribed diseases caused 0.5×10^6 lost days (34). Even if we multiply by ten to allow for non-prescribed diseases, industrial disease, measured in this way, seems a smaller problem than industrial accidents.

Conclusions

This paper has explored, in a preliminary way, the possibility of using estimates of the probability of death for comparing acute and chronic hazards. The purpose of doing so is to help us decide whether reduction of acute risks or reduction of chronic risks should have priority. Results suggest that the allocation of resources between the two types of hazard is probably not too far out.

A major difficulty is knowing whether or not delayed death is worse than immediate death. On the one hand we have 20-40 more years life; on the other hand we have the worry of possible disease and years of illness before death. Perhaps these two effects can be offset and all deaths treated as equally undesirable?

We do need a new look at the data on which TLVs are based in order to estimate (however roughly and with a safety factor to cover uncertainties) the probability of death at various exposures. Until we can do this we do not know if we are setting TLVs too low and thus spending on industrial hygiene resources that would be better spent on the reduction of acute hazards (or vice versa).

However, the evidence suggests that in many industries the acute and chronic risks are now within an order of magnitude of each other. This may not seem very good but is not bad for problems of resource allocation. Nationally, for example, our allocation of resources to medical care, road safety, industrial safety and discouragement of smoking bears no relation at all to either the relative risks or the costs of reducing the hazards (2).

Further work

In this paper the relative sizes of short and long-term risks have been compared and it has been assumed that if we can identify the higher risks, we should give priority to their reduction. There is, however, another way of comparing risks. We can give priority to the expenditure which will save most lives per £1 million spent. I have argued elsewhere (2) that this method should not be preferred as it leads to the toleration of risks which are high but expensive to reduce but that it may be useful as a secondary criterion.

In the present case I have no information on the relative costs of reducing short and long-term risks. This is a subject worthy of further investigation.

Acknowledgements

Thanks are due to the many colleagues who suggested ideas for this paper or commented on the draft. The opinions however are the author's.

References

1. Kletz, T A. I Chem E Symposium Series No 34, p 75, 1975.
2. Kletz, T A. In Chemical Engineering in a Changing World. (ed) W T Koetsier, Elsevier, Amsterdam, 1976.
3. Kletz, T A. Hydrocarbon Processing, 56, 297, 1977.
4. Kletz, T A. Chemical Engineering Progress, 72, 48, 1976.
5. Kletz, T A. Reliability Engineering, 1, 35, 1981.
6. Lees, F P. Loss Prevention in the Process Industries, Butterworths, 1980.
7. Lawley, H G. Chemical Engineering Progress, 72, 45, 1974.
8. Lawley, H G. Reliability Engineering, 1, 89, 1980.
9. Gibson, S B. Chemical Engineering Progress, 72, 59, 1976.
10. Stewart, R M. I Chem E Symposium Series No 34, p 99, 1971.
11. Jacobsen, M et al. In Inhaled Particles. (ed) W H Walton, Unwin Bros. 3.
12. Private communication - a report is being prepared for publication.
13. Lawrence, E. (ed) Annual Abstract of Statistics, Table 2.32. HMSO, 1981.
14. Griffiths, R F. Atom, p 3, December 1970.
15. Kinchin, G H. Proceedings of the Inst of Civil Engineers, Part 1, 64, 431, 1978.
16. Reissland, R and Harris, V. New Scientist, p 809, 13th September 1979.
17. Griffiths, R F. Dealing with Risk. Manchester University Press, 1981.
18. Committee on Hygiene Standards, British Occupational Hygiene Society. Annals of Occupational Hygiene, 11, 47, 1968.
19. Roach, S A. Control limits (workplace environment). National Health and Safety Conference, Victor Green Publications, London, 1980.
20. Human Health and Environmental Toxicants, International Congress and Symposium Series No 17. Royal Society of Medicine, 1980.
21. Mountfield, B A. A behavioural approach to the assessment of risk. MSc Dissertation, London School of Hygiene and Tropical Medicine, September 1978.
22. Fielder, R J. Toxicity Review 4: Benzene. HMSO, 1982.
23. Truhaut R. Am Ind Hyg Ass J, 41, 685, 1980.
24. Baldwin, R H. Chem Tech, 9, 156, 1979.
25. Health and Safety Executive. Health and safety statistics 1978-1979, HMSO, p 12 & 63, 1981.
26. See Reference 22, p 64.
27. The Royal Society. Long-term toxic effects; a study group report. Royal Society, London, 1978.
28. Epstein, S. The politics of cancer. Sierra Club Books, 1979, revised edition, Anchor Press, 1979.
29. National Cancer Institute, National Institute of Environmental Health Sciences and National Institute for Occupational Safety and Health. Estimates of the fraction of cancer in the US related to occupational factors, 1978.
30. ASTMS. The prevention of occuptational cancer: policy document. 1980.
31. Peto, R. Nature, 284, 297, 1980.
32. Workplace Health and Safety Services. TUC publication, 1980.
33. Farmer, D. Health and Safety at Work, p. 18, May 1982.
34. Department of Health and Social Security. Social security statistics. Table 20.70, 1977.

PART 2

Risk From Chemicals

6
Medical priorities - the place of chemicals

ROY GOULDING

First, I must point out - though within a few minutes of hearing what I have to say this should be obvious to you - I am in no position today (or at any other time, for that matter) to present you with a learned discourse packed with science and mathematics and enlivened with an audio-visual accompaniment glittering with risk-benefit calculations.

Instead I am taking the liberty afforded me by the generous attitude of the organisers of this seminar to voice what could easily be a personal and singular point-of-view. My excuse for doing so is that I am still, indeed, a medical practitioner who has found himself engaged over many decades in the realm of toxicology, and of clinical toxicology in particular, so that I can look back over the unfolding events in the past and, at the same time, have the audacity to wonder how they will progress in the future - with especial reference to the survival of mankind and of the social systems in which we presently find ourselves.

In so far as I am still a doctor, my primary concern is with the sick and how to relieve their suffering and distress and how I might profitably prolong their lives. I am not content with back-room research and speculation and less still am I enchanted with the political manipulations of medicine, or theorizing within so-called expert committees that have proliferated throughout the organisations and international agencies of the world.

Instead, I prefer adherence to the principles enunciated by Hippocrates, with the role of the medical man (or woman) being centred on the recognition, diagnosis, treatment and prevention of those diseases that beset the members of the community in which one practises. This, I admit, is an essentially pragmatic approach. After all, the doctor in his surgery, office, or consulting rooms (call it what you will) is not expected by those patients who seek his aid to sit back, however impressively, and expound with erudition on, say, the biochemical and genetic explanations of some pathology, but rather face up to the situation, decide what is wrong and suggest how it might be righted. There is no excuse for selecting just the interesting cases and puting the rest casually aside. In short, he must get on with the task expected of him. Emboldened, as it were, by this philosophy, I would like to spend a little time on the ailments from which people demand relief.

First of all, very few of them want to die. Here the doctor knows that, ultimately, he is going to fail them, for it has been observed, albeit cynically, that there are two inevitables from which there is no escape in

modern society: namely, death and taxation. The latter is beyond the determination of medical skills and so, up to a point, is the former. But what the
doctor sets out to do, I would suggest, is first to defer, so far as he can, the
demise of the individuals in his care for as long as possible - at least beyond
the psalmist's span - and, over the intervening years, to render that life as
healthy as possible, both physically and mentally.

That brings me immediately to a consideration, first, of the principal
causes of death (ie mortality) and, more pertinently, the causes of early
death. Those of you who are here today from other lands (and that distinction, Professor Oliver, I regret applies to Scotland as well) will forgive
me, I hope, if I concentrate on the statistics for England and Wales. That is
not because I chauvenistically dismiss the fate of (dare I say?) 'foreigners',
but because I am more familiar with these and because I am illustrating a
theme. The figures thus collated by the Office of Population Censuses and
Surveys (OPCS) in London happen conveniently to meet my needs. Further,
in order not to aggravate bewilderment by displaying masses of details
upon the screen, I am going to content myself - and I trust you as well - by
approximations, or 'roundings-off', for a measure of imprecision is probably
of little consequence in this context.

Out of a total population of some 49 millions in the territories
under consideration, about 580 000 are registered as dying each year. At first
glance this might infer an inordinate longevity and, as it turns out, many
people do continue to an extraordinary maturity in England and Wales.
What, though, is more arresting, is the realisation that 8000 of these deaths
occur in the first twelve months of life, over 90 000 fail to survive beyond the
age of 60 and, to borrow the psalmist's standard again, 200 000 of them are
dead by 70. In terms of equity, that would appear a little unreasonable. On
the other hand, no less than 380 000 soldier on after 70, but, of course, from
these mortality computations alone I cannot express any opinion about the
quality of life thereafter, or whether it is largely 'sans teeth, sans eyes, sans
everything'. Speaking personally, though, as I advance more closely towards the dividing line my own preoccupation with avoiding nemesis int-
ensifies progressively. Nevertheless, if I am realistic about fate, I should not
be too anxious about these veterans - aside from the domestic, social and
medical provisions made for them - but should direct my interest to the 200
000 who fall short of the ordained target.

At the outset, the OPCS tabulations are informative. Infectious
diseases of all types are responsible for only about 1300 deaths before the
age of 70 and 2200 in all, lending weight to the oft-repeated assertion that,
by the 1980s, this form of illness is well under control.

So next we might take an overall look at the other and principal causes
of death. In order of incidence they may be set out as:

Diseases of the circulatory	290 000	Genito-urinary diseases	8000
system (including 165 000		Diseases of the nervous systems	6500
from ischaemic heart disease)		Endocrine and related disorders	6500
Neoplasia	130 000	Road traffic accidents	6000
Respiratory diseases	83 000	(including motor cycles - 1000)	
Injury and poisoning	20 000	Suicide	4500
(with 4000 due to poisoning)		Falls	4200
Diseases of the digestive system	16 000	Congenital disorders	3500

Demonstrably, the failure of the heart and circulation parades as the 'captain of the men of death'; in other words, the ebbing of the life's blood brings 50 percent of the people in England and Wales to their graves. After that comes neoplasia, or cancer, making up 22 percent, followed by respiratory failure and then, somewhat surprisingly, injury and poisoning. In addition, 6000 deaths annually on the roads are not to be ignored, with about 1000 of them involving motor cycles and, as though destiny is not sufficient, 4500 people take their own lives.

Yet it could be argued, as I have already emphasised, that everyone has to die from something. What is much more critical then, may be the proportion that succumbs, as it were, prematurely. Can we accept once more for this purpose the divide of 70 years? If so, we might arrrange the figures simply for those under 70 and the causes of death may then be listed as:

Diseases of the circulatory system	95 000	Road traffic accidents	4500
(including 57 000 from		Suicide	3500
ischaemic heart disease)		Diseases of the nervous systems	3000
Neoplasia	63 000	Congenital disorders	3000
Respiratory diseases	17 500	Endocrine and related disorders	2500
Injury and poisoning	14 000	Genito-urinary diseases	2000
(with 3000 due to poisoning)		Falls	1000
Diseases of the digestive system	6000		

Interestingly enough, the changes in the order are not very striking, except that diseases of the genito-urinary system take a back seat, as do deaths from endocrine, metabolic and related disorders, while road traffic accidents, suicides and congenital disorders tend to move up.

In the cause of the 'patient-corporate', therefore, it looks as though our emphasis medically should be the same, whether we are intent on staving off death, or whether we are going to intensify our efforts towards the under-70s. Whichever way we regard this choice, there is no denying that, in England and Wales during the latter half of the twentieth century, cardiovascular disease and, notably, the ischaemic form, is exacting an enormous toll. So as a toxicologist I must ponder whether what might be termed the materials of my craft can in any way be blamed for this.

Within the repertoire of poisons there are one or two that have displayed some cardiotoxicity experimentally, but I cannot really believe that they figure at all conspicuously in the everyday British diet or 'life-style', or that any of them set up the kind of degenerative changes that we observe in the human arteries. Indeed, I would aver that toxicology has no part to play in establishing the true aetiology of the disease that claims far more lives among the community than any other. That I must leave, if I can invoke him once more, to Professor Oliver and his associates.

May I have your permission now to defer the second item on the list, not to dismiss it by any means, but because I want to give it fuller consideration subsequently? And that brings me to diseases of the respiratory system. They surely kill a large number of people, though proportionately not so many before the age of 70. Closer scrutiny of the statistics reveals that very few indeed on these fatalities can be directly attributable to occupational exposure, such as pneumoconioses and asbestosis. Looking to the pathologists for guidance here I cannot avoid the belief that the lungs of all of us are subject to almost inexorable degenerative changes, to what might be loosely described as 'wearing out'.

Whether this be so, it is incontestable that the respiratory environment, during life, has a very devastating influence upon pulmonary and bronchial integrity. With the advent of the Clean Air Acts I think we can be gratified with the improvement in the atmosphere communally. There are occasional toxic insults upon the lungs in relation to work - to inadequate hygiene, to carelessness and to accidents, but I think it fair to say that these are rare and that the reports of the Employment Medical Advisory Service in this country would confirm this. No, as someone who confesses to the indulgence from time-to-time in a cigarette or cigar, I cannot side-step the conclusions that the habit of smoking is the major demon in this respect. That you may interpret as a poisonous practice, just as King James I did some three centuries ago, but its curbing calls for a fiscal and educational policy that is beyond the competence of a mere clinical toxicologist.

Next we come to injury and poisoning and here I must face up to my obligations. Even in this secure and precaution-minded western world we manage to sacrifice a deplorable figure of as many as 20 000 people in England and Wales each year to events that, in all conscience, should be preventable. Worse still, nearly three-quarters of these ill-fated souls are under 70 years of age. Putting aside those specifically identified as poisonings, I deny any toxicological responsibility for the rest, other than very indirectly in one or two instances. For the sake of human welfare I feel strongly that this feature of mortality upon the escutcheon of public health demands more vigour in its effacement and, in passing, might register my surprise that, in the annual report of the Chief Medical Officer 'On the State of the Public Health for the Year 1982', this topic fails to gain so much as a mention.

As for the actual poisonings, with 4000 deaths a year to our discredit and some 3000 of them involving the under-70s, there is no denying that, if every one of the toxic agents could be completely safeguarded, no one would die from them. But that is manifestly impracticable. Admittedly, more could still be done to obviate the toxic accidents, though these constitute a quite small share of all the poison deaths. From my own experience in the Poisons Unit, verified by other workers similarly engaged elsewhere, I remain convinced that the great majority of those people in this country, just as in most of the other, so-called, developed lands, that meet their ends by poisoning have contrived to do so wilfully by their own hands. Fundamentally this is a personal and social malaise, disposed to alleviation only politically, psychologically and socially, to which process the toxicologist, as such, has little to subscribe.

On the fatal disease of the digestive system it is difficult to generalise, for they range over such an extraordinary wide range of pathological entities. I may be proved wrong, but as I work my way down the tabulation of causes, I alight on hardly any that I would designate as of toxic aetiology, with the exception of alcoholic cirrhosis of the liver (which reassuringly, is of minor incidence in England and Wales).

Then we reach road traffic accidents which dispose of some 6000 victims each year, with 3500 of them under 70 and about 1000 of them being motor-cyclists. Alcohol and, in some measure, drugs could be implicated in some of these, but the findings suggest that these are not major factors.

Rather would I submit that what is more to blame herein is the quest for speed, the promotional encouragement blatantly accorded this by the car manufacturers' promotion techniques and the apparently utter incapability of the police to enforce speed limits.

With regard to suicides, the same comments apply as to poisonings, with which they are inter-related.

Diseases of the nervous system are not a major cause of death and with these it is difficult to assess the extent to which toxic agents might play a part. There is a diversity of diagnostic headings and it is conceivable that some of the hereditary and degenerative disorders have a toxic background - Wilson's disease, for instance, as well as certain of the peripheral neuritides and cerebral/cerebellar disorders, as from arsenic, lead, mercury and so on, but questionable whether say, multiple sclerosis, epilepsy, motor neurone disease, myasthenia gravis, etc. could have the same inculpation. Not that we should be too dismissive about this for, as you are aware, we are still struggling to elucidatethe aetiology of that ghastly neuro-muscular disease that afflicted a large number of the Spanish population, apparently from a toxic component in a consignment of rape seed oil sold as a foodstuff.

Before I delve any further among the minor causes of death I must return to neoplasia, or cancer. You will not need reminding that this is pleomorphic and can arise initially within almost any organ in the body. It can be rampant, or virtually indolent. Histologically it may take on different guises. Some forms respond to treatment, surgically or medically; others are quite resistant. It is known, albeit infrequently, to regress spontaneously. Overall its incidence progresses with advancing years, though particular types are more characteristic of childhood. So, I would suggest that we should never speak of cancer, in the singular, but of neoplasia, or cancers in the plural.

We may note that over recent years some progress in treatment has been achieved, but this is minimal and disappointing overall. That is why the emphasis has shifted to prevention. Yet, notwithstanding the vast amounts of money and scientific intellect applied to the subject there is still no convincing explanation of the mechanism of carcinogenesis. Infection, with particular reference to viruses, has been highlighted. Changes in the immunological status of the organism have been entertained. Oncogenes are now being explored and the ubiquitous presence of the superoxide ion and its corresponding relationship to the enzyme superoxide dismutase has become fashionable. Steadfastly throughout, moreover, the idea has been exalted that fundamentally neoplasia begins with mutagenesis and, by this theory, simple tests in the pattern of those eponymously linked with Ames have become almost a gospel.

Unashamedly I borrow from an address delivered by Dr Philip Handler of the US National Academy of Sciences to the North Western University Cancer Center, for he expresses my own scepticism more trenchantly than ever I could do myself. It is curious, for example, that after the putative mutagen gains access to the body as a whole it sets up a neoplastic focus in just one site and, thereafter, the process smoulders for years before announcing itself. It is odd, too, that when cells from a growing teratoma have been introduced into developing embryos at the early blastula stage they proceed to participate in normal development. One could continue in this vein with a whole series of anomalies. My main object though, is to query the validity of the concept that so much cancer is due to chemicals, con-

scious though I am of the hopelessness of someone suffering from a hae-
mangiosarcoma from vinylchloride monomer, or a mesothelioma from asbestos, or a
bladder cancer from an aromatic amine.

Historically I wonder if the wrong route were taken some years ago when
we first designed carcinogenicity screening experiments in animals. As the
medical secretary of what was the first UK Carcinogen Panel I recall the
discussions very well. We chose rodents out of convenience and with little
regard to any analogy they might exhibit with the human. We opted for
heavy dosing schedules, to be sure of getting an effect. Success certainly
came our way. Still more embarassing has been the plethora of positive
results emanating from the bio-assay campaign of the US National Cancer
Institute. That cancer is the product of environmental factors has become
increasingly obvious; that these factors are constituted of much more than
synthetic chemicals alone is only now becoming apparent. You will remember that, with due deference to the sensationalists, there is no
epidemic of cancer and that, when the mortailty figures are age-weighted,
there has been no significant increase in the total incidence of this disease
over the past half-century - during which era the synthetic chemical industry
has burgeoned. Moreover, it has been calculated that, if all cancer were
abolished, then 'the mean age of death of the American population would
increase by only one-and-a-half to two years'.

It is not my remit here today to treat you to a homily on malignant
disease; that would take far too long. But this brief review does bring me to
the gravamen of my presentation. Over the last thirty-or-so years a vast,
new curricular subject, scientific discipline and major industry has mat-
erialised (I choose that last verb advisedly). It embraces the activities of
thousands of qualified scientists throughout the world and absorbs millions
of pounds, or dollars, in expenditure annually. I have in mind toxicology and,
above all, experimental toxicology. Governmental and other authorities
impose obligations in this sphere with the avowed declaration of safe-
guarding the public health. The science itself flourishes within this climate. It
is inventive, too. It is constantly devising new techniques which, once
launched, no one has the courage to put aside. So a mammoth undertaking
is under way and gathering pace and power.

I would not deplore this, if only we could draw upon unlimited
resources. Nevertheless, when medically I contemplate the whole vista of
human disease and discomforture, I have a feeling that we are not really
doing our best for what I have called the 'patient-corporate'. In the beginning of my talk I was at some pains to set out the principal causes of death,
particularly those making their impact before the age of 70. Now I would like
to recall the morbidity with which the general practitioner has to contend,
again with grateful acknowledgement to the OPCS. Expressed as what are
entitled patient 'contacts', or patient 'episodes', these impose themselves in
the following order:

    1. Respiratory diseases
    2. Cardio-vascular disorders
    3. Mental problems
    4. Nervous or sensory disorders
    5. Musculo-skeletal complaints.

Can we honestly believe that all this toxicological testing and experimentation is doing very much towards coping with the medical ills that beset our society? I have not forgotten the theme of this meeting is risk-benefit. I am, therefore, simply pondering whether the risks entailed by curtailing some of these toxicological excesses would not be substantially outweighed by the benefits to be derived from more resolutely tackling the diseases which are the everyday burden of patient and doctor alike.

Hereabouts you may well dispute my thesis. You may well argue that it is just the performance of all this toxicity testing that has brought about the admirable state of affairs by which, as I have emphasised, we are spared the worst depredations and excesses of chemical poisoning. Let me, then, make myself clear. I am not advocating the total abandonment of animal testing. My worry about experimental toxicology, though, is that today it has become a powerful religion, which few have the temerity to disavow. And, like other religions, it flourishes on a creed, rather than on reason. Its prelates are the regulatory toxicologists, both on committees and on staff, whose pronouncements are doctrinal and must never be questioned and, like all high priests, they infuse their duties with a sense of self-righteousness. Yet if you pause to read their sermon in the recent Royal Society publication on Risk Assessment you will observe that, when they are honest with themselves, they are in disarray.

Will you allow me a brief postscript? Toxicology unfortunately lends itself to political polarisation, expressed as the innocent, exploited public and the workers on the one hand and the multinational capitalist corporations inspired by cupidity on the other. The media and the politicians have not been slow to fashion these opposing concepts to their own ends. We have witnessed this even in the present seminar. May I then conclude by quoting again from Philip Handler: 'Scientists best serve public policy by living within the ethics of science, not those of politics', though I would propose here that, in this context, doctors should equally be the subject of this declaration, as scientists in general.

May I end, as I began, on a personal note? I am neither very God-fearing, nor an anti-vivisectionist. My worry, though, is that if, ere long, I should be summoned in front of my Creator to give an account of myself on earth will I be able, as a medical doctor with the professional obligations attached thereto, at once to excuse myself for condoning the sacrifice of so many of His smaller creatures whilst apparently disregarding the more obvious sickness, suffering and early death that overtakes so many patients? I doubt it.

7

Risk of correcting risks of cardiovascular disease by drugs

M F OLIVER

The two principal risk factors for the development of coronary heart disease (CHD) and strokes are raised blood pressure and raised blood cholesterol, or cholesterol-containing lipoproteins. Drugs which enable the medical profession to reduce blood pressure and reduce blood cholesterol levels are now widely available and more are being developed year by year. Their use in primary prevention means advising that the appropriate drug should be taken on an indefinite basis, but there are two problems which must be resolved before such advice is implemented.

One is what is the actual risk and who is really at risk? If the relationship between a risk factor and disease is strong and clearly a linear one, then it is appropriate to apply preventive measures to all of the population so as to reduce the risk of everyone - this applies to cigarette smoking and CHD. If there is a curvi-linear and less strong relationship between the risk factor and disease - as exists between serum cholesterol and CHD or blood pressure and stroke - there is little to be gained from lowering the level of the risk factor below the threshold where the relationship becomes weak and non-existent. If there is a J- or U- relationship between the risk factor and disease, then it is obvious that it would be unwise to lower the risk factor in any section of the population other than those with relatively marked elevation: this applies to blood pressure and CHD.

The other problem is that we are now confronted with the possibility that the risk of correcting risk by indefinite use of some drugs might be greater than the uncorrected risk. Also, there is a paradox in that it is only certain whether any of the drugs are safe for long-term use after they have been given for many years. For each we have to go through a learning period and have to try out their safety.

Quite clearly, it would be unethical not to intervene in those with maximum risk for cardiovascular diseases and there should be no argument in such individuals - eg, top 5th percentile - about the use of drugs even when they carry a degree of risk themselves. The unresolved question is to what extent drugs should be given on an indefinite basis in the upper 60-95% of the population who have only a mild or moderate increase in risk.

What then is the actual risk of CHD and strokes in relation to raised blood pressure and raised serum cholesterol? In the US Pooling Project comprising 5 core studies of 8422 men aged 40-64, 11% with serum cholesterol greater than 269 mg/dl and 10% with systolic blood pressure (SBP) 144-157 mmHg and/or diastolic blood pressure (DBP) of 92-97 mmHg developed CHD over the next 8.6 years. Even compounding these risk factors with cigarette smoking and age, the maximum 8.6 year CHD risk for men aged 55-59 was only 22%. The estimated risk of CHD over the 25 years age span of 40 to 64 years is 32% for the top quintile of serum cholesterol and 34% for that of SBP or DBP. Even lower estimates of risk were derived from the Whitehall Civil Servants Study of 18 403 men aged 40-64.

Similarly, while the risk of strokes is increased with raised blood pressure, the actual 10 year risk in those with moderate hypertension (DBP 95-104 mmHg) is only 7% of men and 4% of women (40-49) and 9% of men and 7% of women (50-59).

Thus, the majority apparently at risk will not develop CHD or a stroke in the foreseeable future and, if drugs are to be used for modifying the CHD or stroke risk by treating mild or moderate hypercholesterolaemia or hypertension, most will receive such drugs unnecessarily.

This might be acceptable if the available drugs were safe. But this is far from the case. For example, clofibrate is associated with an increase in non-cardiovascular mortality; triparanol (MER-29) led to baldness and cataract. Beta-blockers reduce mental anxiety in many and cause lethergy, cold extremities and dreams. They affect serum lipoproteins adversely. Diuretics increase the prevalence of male impotence, arrhythmias and gout and cause hypokalaemia-hypomagnesaemia. Some oral hypoglycaemic drugs increase the incidence of myocardial infarction.

In general, pharmaceutical companies undertake extensive and scrupulous screening tests of a new drug in numerous animal species (and toxicity is often tested at concentrations many times in excess of that which will be given to humans). They demonstrate their effectiveness in altering a given measurement in man, such as blood pressure in patients with raised blood pressure, and only as a consequence of these careful tests will the Committee on Safety of Medicines and the Food and Drug Administration of the USA license the product. But, the licences are usually granted on the basis that the drug has not been shown to be toxic to animals, that it has not produced any 'nasty' effects in orthodox biochemical or haematological tests, that it produces no side effects when given over a few months to man and that it continues to be effective in the short-term in correcting the abnormal measurement at which it is aimed. What the drug might do to the metabolism of the body when given over years and the extent to which it is safe can only be identfied when it is actually given over many years to a large number of people.

This demands large-scale clinical trials to prove safety as much as efficacy. Most of the adverse effects mentioned would not have been identified in the absence of a clinical trial. The increasing pressures to use drugs for primary prevention without prior clinical trial is unethical and irresponsible. The problem is a unique one for the end of this century.

We have never seen such widespread prescription usage of drugs by healthy individuals in the community and we have no comprehensive monitoring systems which permit us to look at the repercussions or to provide adequate data to enable responsible decisions to be taken for or against specific intervention. It is relatively easy to be alerted to an expected side effect or even to something obvious like a skin rash or jaundice. But it is the insidious, such as fatigue in the case of beta-blockers, or the unexpected, such as male impotence in the case of diuretics that takes time - and many tragic cases - for recognition: such developments will not appear through the yellow card system.

Death certificates are useless in that they do not provide any information about prior drug treatment. Post-marketing surveillance by pharmaceutical companies is sketchy. One can be cynical about this and say that it would obviously not be to the advantage of pharmaceutical companies to establish a complex and expensive post-marketing surveillance system. But in reality is it not asking more than is reasonable? Would one have expected the manufacturers of clofibrate, for example, to have monitored the development of diseases and deaths in all who took the drug over a 10 year period?

The Government is the chief client of pharmaceutical companies in this country. It should be the responsibility of the Government in conjunction with pharmaceutical companies to establish adequate data banks for drug usage in healthy people. It is not good enough to try to obtain information from prescription usage. All that it would do is to inform us about the total sales for drugs. Prescription data are not programmed to be able to show that a given individual has taken a drug for X years and therefore permit all on this drug to be pooled for analysis of subsequent disease incidence. Nor do they give information about those who do not take the prescribed drug.

Therefore, I make a plea for the establishment of data banks to identify large sections of the population taking specific drugs with a 5, 10 or 15 year follow-up of the problems and incidence of diseases in comparison with a comparable set of the population not taking the drug. I do not think that this will be particularly difficult or expensive in this computer age, although there may be difficulties with regard to confidentiality but these have been overcome in other aspects of computer data storage. The United Kingdom is no different in regard to this deficiency than any other country and none has yet established an adequate system of surveillance. An international agency, such as WHO, might establish a wider monitoring system which would produce results quicker. Only in this way will it be known when the risk of correcting risk is greater than the uncorrected risk.

8

Hazards and risk levels associated with consumer goods

J COLLIN

When I was invited to present to this First International Risk Seminar a paper dealing with the work of the EEC on the risks arising from the use of chemicals in consumer goods, I immediately sought a definition of the word 'risk'. After consulting various encyclopaedic dictionaries, I was struck by the definition that risk is a 'probability of an uncertain event which may cause harm'.

It is held in certain quarters that risk should be non-existent, that is to say the probability should be zero and the event which may cause harm should be known perfectly. I think this is an ideal towards which one may strive, but which is impossible to achieve.

It therefore seems more reasonable to try to reduce the risks inherent in chemicals contained in consumer goods to an acceptable level by exerting influence on the two parameters: probability and uncertainty - in other words, by undertaking scientific studies in order to define as accurately as possible those incidents which could cause harm.

To illustrate this point, I shall refer to three categories of consumer goods in the manufacture of which chemicals play a large part: cosmetic products, foodstuffs and household products.

Cosmetic products
Article 2 of Council Directive 76/768/EEC on the approximation of the laws of the Member States relating to cosmetic products reads as follows: 'Cosmetic products put on the market within the Community must not be liable to cause damage to human health when they are applied under normal conditions of use'. This means that the risk for the consumer must tend towards zero. This is the main purpose of the Directive.

How is an attempt made to achieve it? The answer is by first of all trying to ascertain the harm which chemicals used in the manufacture of cosmetic products might cause. Thus, Article 11 of the Directive requires the Commission to draw up lists of permitted substances more commonly known as 'approved lists', on the basis of the results of the latest scientific and technical research. These lists cover (currently): preservatives, ultra-violet filters, anti-oxidents and hair dyes, all of which are chemical substances which exert certain biological or chemical actions.

The Council has already adopted a list of colouring agents and a list of preservatives and is now examining a list of ultra-violet filters. For its part, the Commission has begun work on the compilation of a list of anti-oxidants and a list of hair dyes. On account of their properties, these substances exert actions which are biological in the case of preservatives and chemical with anti-oxidants; they are therefore liable to cause damage to human health, although at the same time they enhance the safety in use of cosmetics, as seen with preservatives which prevent micro-biological contamination.

In order to determine the harm that these substances might cause in man, there has been compiled for each of them a scientific dossier which sets out, inter alia, their conditions of use in cosmetic products, their chemical and physical characteristics and, most of all, the available toxicological data. This dossier is examined by the competent health authorities of each Member State and by the Commission, which, for its part, is advised by the Scientific Committee on Cosmetology which was set up by a Commission Decision of 19 December 1977. This Committee is composed of leading figures who are highly qualified in fields such as medicine, toxicology, biology, pharmacology, chemistry and other similar disciplines.

One of the first concerns of this Committee was to specify the approach it was going to adopt. The result of its deliberations will be disseminated shortly in the form of 'Notes of guidance for the toxicity testing of cosmetics ingredients'.

By examining the scientific dossier it is possible to make a fairly close estimate of the harm which chemicals used as ingredients in cosmetic products may cause in man. If the potential harm is considerable, the use of the substance in cosmetics is prohibited and the risk is zero. If no harm is apparent from the dossier, the risk is probably very small and the use of the substance in the manufacture of cosmetics is permitted. A more difficult problem is posed by substances for which dossiers indicate the possibility of harmful effects which, for want of a better word, I will describe as minor - an example being an allergic reaction, since allergy is a very individual phenomenon.

In this case the incident which will cause harm is known. Should the use of the substance in cosmetic products therefore be banned? Opinions are divided. Some agree, because cosmetics are not a vital necessity. Others disagree, on the grounds that it would not be logical to deprive the whole population of a product if the harm concerns only a few people.

The second opinion is the one which has prevailed as far as cosmetics are concerned. However, in this case the risk has been reduced by the probability factor, since the probability of occurrence of the event which causes harm has been diminished by means of labelling and warnings. On the labels of certain cosmetics can be found mandatory warnings such as :
'Can cause allergic reactions, contains ....' or 'Not to be used for babies!'
(If the cosmetic product contains a chemical which is harmful only to babies.)

Foodstuffs
Foodstuffs can contain chemicals which have either been deliberately added (eg colouring agents, preservatives, anti-oxidants, emulsifiers, gelling agents, stabilizers) or have entered the food as a result of contamination of the environment (eg pesticides, heavy metals, toxins).

Since food is ingested, it is necessary to ascertain the dose of such chemicals which might produce a harmful effect - everything is toxic yet nothing is toxic - it is the dose which makes the poison. The toxicological dossier on each substance is examined by the national authorities and by the Commission, which receives advice from the Scientific Committee for Food set up in 1974 and composed of highly qualified experts.

In 1980, this Committee published a document entitled 'Guidelines for the Safety Assessment of Food Additives'. The Committee has adopted the same approach as the joint panels of experts of the World Health Organization (WHO) and the Food and Agriculture Organization (FAO). For certain substances which may be incorporated in foodstuffs - whether or not intentionally - (additives; pesticide residues and contaminants), it specifies acceptable daily intakes (ADIs) - ie quantities of substances, expressed as mg/kg of body weight, which a person may absorb daily throughout his or her life without any harmful effect on health. In those cases where toxicological data are not complete, a provisional ADI is fixed: in certain cases (that of the heavy metals, for example), provisionally tolerable weekly intakes are fixed. Once these intakes have been established, it is possible to specify the tolerance limits in foodstuffs on the basis of the average quantity of the foods consumed by a population.

Recently, in France, an inventory of food quality was drawn up. This inventory provides a great deal of information on the quantities of the various contaminants in French people's food. In the light of these data and of the ADIs, Professor Truhaut concluded that, generally speaking, the substances contained in the food of the French people did not appear to endanger their health. Nevertheless, in the case of certain contaminants such as sulphites in wines and aflatoxins in dried fruit, surveillance must be continued. The purpose of these studies is to ascertain with reasonable certainty the event which may cause damage.

But all these long and difficult studies can never warrant an assumption of zero risk. Certain additives which have been beneficial to health in general may produce side-effects in some people. This is the case with allergic or hypersensitivity reactions. The risk can be lessened by taking measures which will reduce the probability of occurrence of the event, such as informing consumers of the composition of foodstuffs.

The Scientific Committee for Food has always urged that the list of ingredients should appear clearly and correctly on foodstuff labels. This is the principal aim of Council Directive 79/112/EEC on the approximation of the Laws of the Member States relating to the labelling, presentation and advertising of foodstuffs for sale to the ultimate consumer. It is to be regretted, however, that in the case of certain ingredients this Directive allows Member States that so desire to have the labels inscribed with generic designations instead of with specific names.

Household products

The EEC's work in the field of household products is still in its infancy. These consumer goods constitute a special case since in order to do their job, they need to contain reactive and, I might even say, aggressive chemicals. It will therefore inevitably be necessary to accept a certain risk. At the present stage, I can only give you an indication of the Commission's intentions.

The competent departments of the Commission are preparing a proposal for a Council directive on the approximation of the laws, regulations and administrative provisions of the Member States relating to the classification, packaging and labelling of dangerous preparations. All household products to which the definition of a dangerous preparation applies will come within the scope of the directive. Since, from the outset, a risk is accepted, an attempt will be made to reduce it to an acceptable level by :

(i) stating the risk by means of appropriate labelling danger symbols, phrases describing special risks inherent in the use of the product and phrases giving precautionary advice on its use;

(ii) and possibly by enacting provisions governing certain categories of household products, so as to reduce the probability of accidents.

A number of measures are being considered. I shall quote a few examples:

- requiring precise directions for use which can easily be understood by the consumer and which might include precautions to be taken for the storage of the product, destruction of the empty container, etc.

- the inclusion on the labels of such phrases as :'Keep out of the reach of children!' 'Do not pour into other containers which usually contain foodstuffs or beverages!'

- stipulating that the packages must not be attractive to children and that they must be different from those commonly used for foodstuffs

- prescribing a child-resistant closure

- considering the provision of a labelling device denoting danger which can be recognized by the blind.

In regard to the last two items, the Commission is participating in the work of the International Organization for Standardization (ISO) and the European Committee for Standardization (CEN) and could refer to the standards laid down by those bodies.

Finally, and still with the aim of reducing the probability of accidents, the Commission is going to study the possibility of launching a consumer information and education campaign on the risks to which household products can give rise and on the means of preventing them. Too many accidents which happen to children under five years of age, who cannot read labels, are still due to the negligence of adults.

I have tried to show by means of these three examples that the risk due to consumer products can be reduced to an acceptable level both by precise knowledge of events (acquired from scientific studies) and by measures to reduce the probability of occurrence of the incident which can cause the damage, in spite of the fact that the number of chemical substances present in our environment is continually increasing.

I think that proper education and better consumer information could further improve the safety in use of consumer goods. An effort has yet to be made in this field, and the consumer associations are likely to have a major role to play.

9
Extrapolation of risk from low-potency animal carcinogens

F J C ROE

In this paper I shall be concerned with extrapolation from animals to man, only a little with low dose to high dose and from *in-vitro* to *in-vivo*, and not at all with animal models which I regard as largely within the realm of science fiction. Accordingly, it behoves me to start this paper by discussing the meaning of 'animal carcinogen'.

'Animal carcinogen'
This term has been widely used during recent years. Therefore, I accepted its use in the title to this paper. However, I do not regard it as fully meaningful. The term is applied to chemicals, or other agents, for which there is, according to somebody's judgement which may be at fault, acceptable evidence of carcinogenicity, in laboratory animals as distinct from human animals. Of course everyone thinks he knows how to define the term 'carcinogen'. In reality this is not so. Even experts cannot agree. Thus when the Committee on Carcinogenesis of the DHSS in the UK (1) recently set about drawing up guidelines for carcinogenicity testing, the members were unable to agree a definition. Consequently, the term remains undefined. The problem is that broad definitions are of little value and narrow definitions make unacceptable assumptions about mechanisms.

An example of a broad definition would be 'an agent which enhances the age-standardised risk of the development of neoplasia'. The difficulty is that we know of many laboratory situations wherein the incidence of neoplasms can be modified in either direction quite non-specifically - for inst ance, by overfeeding or increasing the proportion of fat in the diet. Consequently, direct extrapolation to man based on such a simple and broad definition leads to all sorts of difficulties.

Davis et al (2) tried to produce lung tumours in female rats by exposing them to tobacco smoke by inhalation. The main finding was a significantly reduced incidence of mammary tumours in the smoke-exposed rats as compared with sham-exposed controls and not, as one might have expected, an increased incidence of lung tumours (Table 1). Mindless extrapolation from this observation would lead one to the conclusion, not that women should refrain from smoking because of risk of lung cancer, but that women should be encouraged to smoke as a protection against cancer of the breast.

Table 1. *Effects of life-time exposure of female Wistar rats to cigarette smoke*
(from Davis et al. Reference 2)

	No. of rats	Squamous tumours of lung		Mammary tumours	
		O+	E*	O+	E*
Smoke exposed	408	4	4.4	37	55.6
Sham exposed	102	0	1.1	40	29
p <			N.S.		0.01

+Observed
* Expected based on age-standardized incidence in the whole study which included 3 other groups.

Simple extrapolation from the study by Dalbey et al (3) on the effects of exposing female rats to cigarette smoke would pose far more problems than it solved (Table 2).

Clearly, no broad definition of the term 'carcinogen' provides a reliable basis for extrapolation to man. So, unless we can identify some other basis, it will be nonsensical to attempt to distinguish between 'high-potency' and 'low-potency' animal carcinogens.

Very commonly in carcinogenicity studies in laboratory animals, particularly on drugs which directly or indirectly affect hormonal status, treatment is associated with increased incidence of some kinds of neoplasm and decreased incidence of other kinds of neoplasm. Overall, there may be little difference between treated and control groups in the expectation of their developing neoplasms at any body site (ie all sites considered together). The fact that the risk of just one kind of neoplasm is enhanced has in the past been enough to result in an agent being dubbed 'an animal carcinogen'. The results of a rat study on reserpine serve as an example (4). In this study groups of 50 male and 50 female Fischer rats were fed on diets containing 0, 5 or 10 ppm reserpine for 2 years. In males treatment was

Table 2. *Effect of exposure of female F344 rats to smoke from 7 or 10*
cigarettes per day on % tumour incidence (from Dalbey et al. Reference 3)

	Control (n=93)	Smoke exposed (n=110)
Respiratory tract	1	9*
Mouth	0	5
Dermal sarcoma	0	21*
Pituitary	32*	9
Uterus and ovaries	23*	3
Lymphoid system	33*	10
Mammary glands	16	10
Any tumour at any site	85	68

* p< 0.05

56

associated with a significantly increased incidence of adrenal medullary tumours and a significantly reduced incidence of pituitary tumours (see Table 3).

Table 3. *NCI Study on reserpine in groups of F344 rats*

| | Males | | | | Females | |
	Control	Low dose	High dose	Control	Low dose	High dose
Phaeochromo-cytoma	3	18***	24***	1	3	4
Pituitary adenoma	17	13	6***	21	27	28
Mammary fibroadenoma				14	18	14

*** p = 0.001
** p = 0.01

The authors of the report concluded on this evidence 'Reserpine was carcinogenic for male rats' and even went on to speculate that it might also have proved carcinogenic for female rats had higher doses been tested. They did not discuss the suitability of a model system in which more than a third of the control animals of both sexes developed pituitary tumours, nor did they think to mention that treatment had a beneficial effect on the incidence of these tumours in males.

It is my view that before one even starts to think about extrapolating from laboratory studies to man it is essential to distinguish between three different phenomena, namely, genotoxic carcinogenicity, non-genotoxic carcinogenicity and pseudocarcinogenicity.

It is not always easy to distinguish between these phenomena, particularly because one and the same chemical agent may act in all three ways in the same experimental study or a pseudocarcinogenic or a non-genotoxic carcinogenic effect in an *in-vivo* study may seem to validate a false positive result in an *in-vitro* test for possible genotoxic carcinogenicity. In Table 4 I define these three types of carcinogenicity.

Table 4. *Definitions of three different forms of carcinogenicity*

Genotoxic carcinogenicity: Enhancement of age-standardized risk of development of any type of neoplasm (benign or malignant) at any site, by *a genotoxic* mechanism in *normal* animals (or humans)

Non-genotoxic carcinogenicity: Ditto, but by a non-genotoxic mechanism.

Pseudocarcinogenicity: Enhancement of age-standardized risk of tumour development by a non-genotoxic mechanism in *abnormal* animals

Genotoxic carcinogenicity
In an attempt to overcome these problems, there has been a trend in recent years to distinguish between genotoxic (initiating) and non-genotoxic (promoting) carcinogens. In the case of the former the assumption is made that any agent which damages DNA directly or which gives rise to a metabolite which does so is capable of initiating cancer. This assumption is probably not correct, but it may be difficult to refute in the case of any particular substance. In any case, an important difficulty is that many of the simple test systems for detecting DNA-damaging activity (eg the Ames test using various laboratory strains of *Salmonella typhimurium*) involve bringing the test agent and/or its metabolities into direct contact with virtually naked DNA in a way that may never happen in real life.

Consequently, although there is undeniably a fairly strong positive correlation between genotoxicity as revealed by such tests and demonstrable carcinogenicity, several important false positives are now well recognised. The distinction between true and false positive is both difficult and expensive. It involves undertaking further and increasingly costly tests for gene mutation and chromosome damaging potential, firstly using mammalian cells rather than bacteria and secondly looking for these effects in intact animals. Although tests in animals are clearly more realistic than test-tube tests on bacteria, they are arguably less sensitive. Consequently, there is more than one way of interpreting the combination of a positive result in an *in vitro* bacterial system and a negative result in an *in vivo* system. For this reason, Regulatory Authorities are apt to require negative results in a battery of tests for genotoxicity before they will accept that a positive result in, say, an Ames test is probably false.

If it is clear from the structure of a chemical agent or from a knowledge of its metabolism that it is electrophilic or is metabolised *in vivo* to electrophiles capable of damaging DNA, or if the results of tests for genotoxicity are convincingly positive, then the usual assumption is that there is unlikely to be any threshold for its genotoxic activity. A parallel is drawn between electrophilic chemical agents and ionizing radiation in this regard. In the case of carcinogenesis from penetrating ionizing radiation, there is abundant evidence that the dose-response curve probably passes through the zero exposure point.

It is argued, the same is probably true for electrophilic chemicals. In fact the parallelism is over-stated. Many highly electrophilic chemicals have no 'penetrating' ability. They react with the first protein they come across and may never reach any cellular DNA let alone tissues distant from the point of first contact. Some of the false positives seen in bacterial mutagenicity systems may be explicable in this way. Also, it is easy to understand that chemically highly reactive electrophilic agents may in practice be far less dangerous than less active agents.

One of the greatest advances in cancer research was the recognition that apparently unreactive chemicals may be converted into electrophilic metabolites by normally present body enzymes - by a process known as *metabolic activation*. There is little obvious parallel between genetic damage by penetrating ionizing radiation and genetic damage due to chemical agents which are only genotoxically active after metabolic activation. For the latter type of agent to cause DNA damage it has to reach a site where the required metabolising enzymes are active.

Most ingested chemicals pass via the portal vein to the liver - a site of abundant metabolic activity. It is therefore not surprising that the liver is a common site for tumour development when animals are exposed to chemicals which can give rise to electrophilic metabolites. For some such chemicals the liver acts as a protective screen for other potentially vulnerable tissues. However, this defensive screen can be overwhelmed by excessive exposure so that at high but not low doses the risk of tumour development at other body sites is increased. These considerations justify the expectation that there may be thresholds for some genotoxic carcinogens. Also, coupled with the fact that the liver is a target for a high proportion of so-called animal carcinogens, the fact that in Europe and North America liver cancer in humans is both rare and not increasing, provides considerable assurance that people in these countries are not consuming large or increasing amounts of genotoxic carcinogens.

In the course of my work in connection with the safety evaluation of drugs, food constituents, food additives and other environmental chemicals, I encounter far more examples of non-genotoxic carcinogenicity and pseudocarcinogenicity than of genotoxic carcinogenicity. Therefore, in my opinion it is never sensible just to assume that an increase in incidence of one or other kind of tumour in an animal test is a manifestation of genotoxic carcinogenicity. Evidence of genotoxicity should be actively sought. On the other hand, my views are in accord with conventional prudence when it comes to assessing possible risk to man from proven or probable genotoxic carcinogens. Thus, I agree with the view that no threshold should be assumed unless the mechanism underlying the operation of such a threshold has been identified.

Non-genotoxic carcinogens
For me, non-genotoxic carcinogenicity is a far more interesting, challenging and important subject than genotoxic carcinogenicity. Some investigators who use the term 'non-genotoxic carcinogenesis' or 'epigenetic carcinogenesis' regard them as synonymous with 'tumour promotion'. I disagree As I see it, there are numerous quite different, and sometimes quite complex, non-genotoxic mechanisms which may operate to increase cancer risk. Indeed, I believe that progress in understanding carcinogenesis is being seriously held up by those who assume that all non-genotoxic carcinogens act like TPA, the phorbol ester which promotes skin tumour development following subcarcinogenic exposure of mouse skin to a known carcinogen.

Alternative mechanisms include immune-suppression, viral activation, and enzyme induction. However, most important of all, I believe, is disturbance of hormonal status. Until a decade or so ago, the average medical student would have ended his training being aware of the existence of only a relatively short list of major hormones which are released into the blood stream by easily recognisable endocrine glands. In recent years there has been an explosive increase in knowledge concerning growth-regulatory substances and homeostatic controlling mechanisms. Numerous neurocrine and paracrine hormones have been identified and disturbances of their secretion and action are now known to be associated with an increasing number of diseases in animals and man. So far this burgeoning knowledge has been largely ignored by investigators in the field of environmental carcinogenesis and by Regulatory Authorities responsible for interpreting the results of animal studies.

Also, for example, substance X which is commonly present in food consumed by humans. Before I tell you what substance X is, let me tell you what happened to male rats when they were exposed to it in the diet. Introduction of 20% of X into the diet was associated with significantly increased incidences of tumours of the testis and adrenal medulla but a reduced incidence of islet cell tumours of the pancreas (see Table 5)

Now let me tell you that X was nothing other than the sugar of mothers' milk, namely lactose. It surely is interesting to speculate that if

Table 5. *Effects of feeding X on % of male rats with certain tumours*

Tumour type	Control	Treated
Testis - Leydig cell	4	24**
Adrenal medulla		
- benign or malignant	20	42*
- malignant	6	18*
Pancreas - islet cell	14*	2

* p = 0.005
** p = 0.01

these data had emerged from an NCI Bioassay study, the report would have concluded 'Lactose was carcinogenic for male rats, in which it caused tumours of the testis and adrenal gland'. I doubt whether anyone has been foolish enough to test lactose for genotoxicity but assuming that the *in vivo* data are manifestations of non-genotoxic carcinogenicity, what is the mechanism? I suspect that research in the field of peptide hormones will soon give us the answer.

A probably important clue to the mechanism lies in the effect of high dietary levels of lactose on the absorption of calcium from the gut in rats. In the gut, lactose is hydrolysed to glucose and galactose. The latter is only relatively slowly absorbed in the small intestine. As a consequence, some of the monosaccharide reaches the large bowel and caecal enlargement becomes evident. Now, it seems that calcium is absorbed along with monosaccharides and, in lactose-fed rats where sugars are being absorbed not only throughout the small intestine but in the large bowel as well, the overall absorption is advantageous to young growing mammals that need calcium to build their bones. The enhancement of calcium absorption in rats by high dietary levels of lactose can be so pronounced that it causes various kinds of nephrocalcinosis.

The activity of many endocrine glands is dependent in some way on calcium. In the case of the adrenal medulla, hypocalcaemia due to vitamin D deficiency is associated with decreased catecholamine output. Correction of the hypocalcaemia by dietary administration of lactose without additional vitamin D restores adrenal functioning to normal (5). Maybe an excessive absorption of calcium acts as a stimulus for the adrenal medulla to proliferate although the curious thing is that the phaeochromocytomas that arose in lactose-fed rats were chromaffin negative, that is to say they, were non-functional.

The rat appears to be somewhat unique both in its response to high levels of dietary lactose and in its propensity to develop non-functional tumours of adrenal medulla. By comparison with the rat the evidence that lactose increases the calcium absorption in man is neither extensive nor convincing. Also there is no evidence that hypercalcaemia is associated with proliferative changes in the adrenal medulla in humans (6).

With lactose then we have a striking example of non-genotoxic carcinogenesis. Lactose is non-genotoxic and, in the rat, the effects on the adrenal medulla and testis have only been seen when high dietary levels have been fed over long periods. The type of adrenal tumour that arises in rats is quite common in untreated rats but is exceptionally rare in man. The mechanism by which lactose enhances adrenal medullary tumour risk although not fully elucidated is probably not operative in man. In the present state of our knowledge it would be utterly nonsensical to attempt to calculate from these rat data, cancer risk to man by the use of a mathematical model.

Pseudocarcinogenicity
The sad and sorry truth is that man has not yet mastered the problem of keeping experimental animals throughout their lives such that they remain in normal health. Of course great strides have been made in the field of infectious and parasitic disease, so that epizootics of diseases such as ectromelia in mice and progressive chronic respiratory disease in rats are largely a phenomena of the past. However, the elimination of these diseases has resulted in the recognition of, and possibly the actual enhancement of, a variety of conditions which are obviously laboratory artefacts. The full list of such artefacts, which during my work as a histopathologist I come upon almost every day, is horrendous.

During the past year I have seen, in two separate studies, in control and treated animals alike very high incidences of severe retinal atrophy due to over-exposure to quite ordinary levels of fluorescent light.

In another study, I have seen skin lesions of the foot pads and tails in most animals because they were housed in cages with unsuitably designed metal grids. In addition I have seen high incidences of dental root abscesses and degenerative neuropathy of the cauda equina. However most impressive of all are the extraordinarily high incidences of endocrine gland tumours and hormone-associated tumours that many investigators have come to believe as normal for the aged rat - in much the same way as bronchitis was once regarded as normal for the mature Englishman in the days of heavy air pollution.

I began this talk with illustrations of how exposure of rats to tobacco smoke was found to reduce the incidences of various tumours. If we look again at Table 3 we see that arguably the most notable feature of the results was not the fact that smoking reduced the incidence of pituitary, genital tract and lymphoid tumours, but the fact that these tumours occurred in such high incidence in the sham-exposed animals. I suggest to you that the correct interpretation of these results is that the sham-exposed animals were *abnormal* in respect of these tumours and smoke exposure made them *more normal*. The fact that the smoke-exposed animals put on less weight may well be relevant since it is well known that relatively slight diet restriction can drastically reduce the incidence of pituitary, mammary and many other tumours in laboratory rats and mice (7, 8) .

Current practice in the design of carcinogenicity experiments in rodents is to provide them throughout their lives with free access 24 hours per day to diets that are nutritionally excessive in almost every respect. The animals grow obese and sluggish, and manifest all manner of signs of hormonal disturbance. For instance the serum prolactin levels of rats commonly rise to astronomic levels.

For various reasons which I have discussed elsewhere (9) I suspect that the diet restriction acts to normalise animals with respect to hormonal status not simply by reducing calorie intake, but also by stimulating animals to forage for food when faced during a part of each day with an empty food basket. Nevertheless, the quality of the diet is an important determinant of tumour risk. For example, Gellatly reported a more than five-fold increase in liver tumours in mice when he doubled the fat content of their food (10).

It has recently been claimed that the corn oil, commonly used as the vehicle for the administration of test chemicals to rats and mice in studies sponsored by the National Toxicology Programme in the USA, is carcinogenic. It seems that those who made this claim did not realise that the daily introduction of 0.1 ml of oil into the stomach of a 25 g mouse is equivalant on a dose per unit of body weight to a 70 kg man drinking over a quarter of a litre of oil each day.

Extraordinarily high incidences of all sorts of tumours, particularly of endocrine glands and hormone-controlled tissues, are seen in control animals in most present-day carcinogenicity tests. Table 6 illustrates this for control rats in Kociba et al's (11) definitive carcinogenicity study of the

Table 6. *Hormone-associated neoplasms (%) in ad libitum fed untreated control Sprague Dawley rats observed for up to 26 months (86 rats of each sex) (from Kociba et al, Reference 11)*

	Male	Female
Pituitary	31	63
Adrenal - cortex	2	7
medulla	51	8
Thyroid - C-cell	8	8
Parathyroid	0	1
Pancreas - exocrine	33	0
endocrine	16	9
Testis	7	-
Ovary	-	5
Mammary - fibroadenoma		76
gland adenoma	5	12
other		29

herbicide 2,4,5-T. This happened to be in Sprague Dawley rats, but it is true for rats of all strains. Genetic factors play some part in determining which kinds and how many tumours develop but simple environmental factors relating to the day to day husbandry of animals are by comparison far more important. Amongst these, overfeeding is singly probably the most important factor but other factors such as enforced celibacy under conditions of continuous sexual stimulation are also undoubtedly involved.

The message I wish to leave with you is simple and clear. Is it sensible to use for carcinogenicity assessment, animals which are manifestly grossly abnormal with regard to endocrine status? In my opinion neither a treatment-related increase, nor a treatment-related decrease, in the incidence of such tumours in animals that are grossly hormonally abnormal can be meaningfully interpreted. It is for treatment related increases of tumours in such circumstances that I have introduced the term 'pseudocarcinogenicity'.

The data for reserpine which I showed earlier probably fall into this category and, given time, I could provide many other examples.

There is a desperate need for basic research in animal nutrition and husbandry aimed at defining the conditions necessary for maintaining laboratory animals in normal hormonal status until they are old. Armed with such animals it will be much easier to distinguish between genotoxic and non-genotoxic carcinogens. At present this distinction is being blurred - often hopelessly blurred - by pseudocarcinogenic and pseudoanticarcinogenic phenomena due to laboratory artefacts.

Quantitative assessment of risks to man based on the use of mathematical models, has a place only in connection with genotoxic carcinogenicity. For non-genotoxic carcinogenicity and pseuodocarcinogenicity, it has the status of science fiction. It is overdue that we return to the situation wherein mathematics is regarded as the tool of toxicological science and not vice versa.

References

1. Department of Health and Social Security. Guidelines for the testing of chemical for carcinogenicity. Reports on Health and Social Subjects, 1982,*25*, 1-30. HMSO: London.
2. Davis, B R et al. Response of rat lung to inhaled tobacco smoke with or without prior exposure to 3,4-benzpyrene (BP) given by intratracheal instillation. Brit J Cancer, *31*, 469-484, 1975.
3. Dalbey, W E et al. Chronic inhalation of cigarette smoke by F344 rats. J Nat Cancer Inst, *64*, 383-390, 1980.
4. NIH. Bioassay of reserpine for possible carcinogenicity. UA-DHSS Publication No. NIH 80-1749, 1979.
5. Brion, F and Dupuis, Y. Calcium and monamine regulation: role of vitamin D nutrition. Canad J Physiol, *58*, 1431-1434, 1980.
6. Wrong, O.M. personal communication, 1982.
7. Tucker, M J. The effect of long-term food restriction on tumours in rodents. Int J Cancer, *23*, 803-807, 1971.
8. Conybeare, G. Effect of quality and quantity of diet on survival and tumour incidence in outbred Swiss mice. Fd Cosmet Toxicol, *18*, 65-75, 1980.
9. Roe, F J C. Are nutritionists worried about the epidemic of tumours in laboratory animals? Proc Nutr Soc, *40*, 57-65, 1981.
10. Gellatly, J B M. The natural history of hepatic parenchymal nodule formation in a colony of CB7BL mice with reference to the effect of diet. Chapter in 'Mouse Hepatic Neoplasia' (Eds W.H. Butler and P.M. Newberne) Elsevier: Amsterdam,pp. 77-110, 1975.
11. Kociba, R J et al. Results of a two-year chronic toxicity and oncogenic study of rats ingesting diets containing 2,4,5-Trichlorophenoxyacetic acid (2,4,5-T) Fd Cosmet Toxicol, *17*, 205-221, 1979.

PART 3

The Acceptable Risk - Does It Exist?

10
An overview of
the problem

ROBERT P GIOVACCHINI

In the now dimming light of the past, scientists, applying judgement and experience to the results of their laboratory studies, determined if a material or product was safe. Scientists meeting with their colleagues, be they regulatory or academic, discussed their findings and rationale for determining safety. It was assumed, by the general public, that scientists could determine and measure safety. Suddenly, however, it appears that almost everything is unsafe or certainly less safe than we were led to believe. This is a serious problem because each of us as individuals has to decide what is safe with respect to our families as well as ourselves. Should your wife colour her hair? Should you? Should you drive or fly? What should you have for lunch? Do you want that diet drink or should you drink the water? What do you mean by safe?

Several years ago, I defined safe as 'freedom from unreasonable risk of significant injury under reasonable foreseeable conditions of use' (1). This definition accepted the simple fact that nothing is absolutely safe (now termed the zero risk concept). Everything has some risk associated with it. But there are ways of handling situations, chemical or other, in such a manner as to decrease or eliminate the inherent risk associated with them.

The acceptability of a given level of risk is an entirely different matter. Individuals may well disagree on this issue. What is an acceptable risk, and why is it so difficult to make this decision for society as a whole when, it would appear, as individuals we constantly make risk assessments and decisions on a daily basis?

Setting an acceptable societal risk level is difficult because, as scientists, regulators, manufacturers, legislators, media people, consumers or consumer advocates, we each see risk from a different point of view. In some cases, we each re-interpret the scientific facts to fit our own needs even if the data end up comparing apples and oranges. For example, a politician wants his constituents to know that he is protecting them. They should face no risk while he is in office. A health regulator wants to be certain that all the requisite studies have been conducted, or he does not allow the material on the market, because he must be concerned about being criticised before a legislative oversight committee. The media obviously want to report the news, but also want to sell papers or get high ratings by interesting and controversial stories. An attorney is obligated to defend his client's testing as proving the product is harmless. An industry scientist wants to conduct all the proper studies and determine that the product is safe for marketing. An academic scientist, while wanting to obtain the scientific facts, is motivated also by the availability of industry and government grants.

This very pessimistic view is from a speech I gave years ago on what I then called the new scientific disciplines of political, legislative, legal, industrial, grant, media and consumer advocate toxicology. What does one do with all the information coming to us from all these impeccable sources? Years ago, science spoke with only one voice. Today, the same study is interpreted in so many different ways by these various scientific and social disciplines that it is often difficult to realise that everyone is talking about the same study results. What is the truth? The truth is that *nothing* is safe. Everything you do has some risk associated with it.

And that brings us full circle, back to the question what risks we are willing to accept. Today, there is a growing consensus that an acceptable risk level is about one in one million. What does that mean? That means, according to current risk estimates and accident statistics, about one X-ray per year in an approved hospital, 30 diet drinks per year, 40 tablespoons of peanut butter, 30 pints of milk, 20 cans of beer, 1.5 cigarettes, 10 hours flying at 30 000 feet, two days in New York or Boston, six minutes in a canoe, 30 uses of hair dyes, 100 000 uses of lead acetate hair dyes, 50 miles by car, 10 miles by bicycle, and 1000 miles by airplane (2).

Now that we have briefly reviewed the various types of risks that we normally face during our daily lives, some of our occupations, and some of the sports we indulge in, let's see if we can apply this approach to, for example, chemicals. How much risk is acceptable from chemicals, based on the risks we generally tend to assume? Unfortunately, in the case of oncogenic potential, there is one confounding problem. The risk levels for accidental injury or death are based on retrospective data. In the case of oncogenesis, it generally takes from 15 to 20 years for the disease to demonstrate itself, and even then the cause usually cannot be determined. Many of us would not be alive to see the results of a retrospective risk assessment approach for oncogenesis, even if one could be undertaken.

There are basically two main areas involved in risk assessment. They are usually termed (1) determination of risk and (2) evaluation of risk. Determination of risk is subdivided into (a) identification of risk and (b) estimation of risk. Evaluation of risk is also subdivided into (a) aversion of risk and (b) acceptance of risk.

What is risk? I define risk as the chance of getting hurt, losing, failing, or placing one's self in a dangerous or hazardous position. Hazard is when the potential for harm is present. Thus, something is safe when the risk or hazard is acceptable to you.

Toxicologists can identify, screen, measure, monitor and diagnose biological hazard. They can, through appropriate studies, identify biological risk. Percival Pott, in 1775, is credited for being the first to identify, screen, measure, and diagnose cancer of the scrotum as an occupational disease in chimney sweeps in England (3). Science can assess the probabilities and consequences of hazard and risk based upon the facts, assumptions, and statistical extrapolations. We can define conditions of use, the amount of exposure, and the route of exposure; relate exposure concentration to toxicological effects; and assess the probability of toxicological effect to its possible consequences (4,5,6,7).

While not everyone agrees on methods for identifying, measuring, and screening risk, we must find some way to estimate human risk by extrapolating from high dose animal feeding studies, the second step in the determination of risk. There are various techniques available to us when determining risks to carcinogens. They include the linear dose response, the probit model, the single hit, multistage, log-logistic, and multi-hit model. Even today, there is no agreement on which model is the best to use.

The advantage of the log-probit method is its principle that carcinogens give some risk at any exposure level and the use of upper confidence limits. But this method does not fit experimental data too well, and the slope of the dose-response curve becomes very shallow as the dose approaches zero. Thus, this procedure predicts low-dose risks considerably below those of other models (8,9). The single hit model was first used by the radiation toxicologists who conceived the theory that oncogenesis develops when a cell is hit by a threshold level of radiation. The probability of carcinogenesis is then expected to be proportional to the total amount of radiation to which one is exposed over a lifetime. Since this model assumes a linear response in the observed range, it always gives a very low estimate of the safe dose when compared to other models. The same kind of problems are reported with the multi-stage, gamma multi-hit model, and the time to tumour models (10 - 18).

The problem of determining an appropriate model for low dose extrapolation stems from the fact that there is no known threshold dose below which any response is impossible for every single individual. If we use saccharin as an example, we can conclude, using an appropriate statistical model, that the risk of bladder cancer from drinking soft drinks that contain saccharin varies from 0.22 to 1 144 000 cases of bladder cancer over the next 70 to 80 years. When the FDA reviewed the question of aflatoxins in peanuts and corn, it found that, if it used a conservative statistical method and extrapolated results directly from rat studies to humans, the statistical estimates of lifetime liver cancer rates exceeded the lifetime liver cancer rate from all causes in the United States (19,20).

How can we have such disparate results when we apply statistical techniques to the animal data for extrapolation to a human risk factor? Hutt has probably answered the question as well as it can be answered. He states that there are five obstacles to reasoned scientific decision making on safety issues:

> First, the scientific data base is seldom adequate to make a definitive safety judgement on any substance; second, even when substantial safety data are available there is seldom scientific agreement on the meaning or significance of that information; third, even assuming that an adequate scientific data base were available, together with scientific agreement on the meaning and significance of that data, there appears to be no public or scientific concensus today on the risk, or on the uncertainty, acceptable to justify the marketing of any substance for public use; fourth, there is enormous and continuing public pressure for governmental agencies to resolve whatever may be the latest current safety issue promptly and decisively; and fifth, regardless of the outcome of the decision, those who disagree with it will continue to pursue the matter through all available channels, while those who agree with it inevitably will remain silent, preparing themselves for the next issue. (21)

As stated earlier, evaluation of risk is divided into two components. They are, one, the aversion of risk, and two, the acceptance of risk. Also, let us not forget the fact that some risks are voluntary while others are involuntary. We decide to drive a car, to smoke, to drink, to fly, to attend a meeting, to ski. However, if we are breathing polluted air, drinking polluted water, or eating contaminated food or a meteor or a space craft falls on us, we have no decision in, or in some cases had no knowledge of, the risks involved. This second part of the risk assessment decision tree takes us into the area of social and philosophical concepts where everyone can be an expert. How much risk are you willing to take? How much risk are the rest of us willing to allow you to take? Can we reach a consensus on what is an acceptable risk?

It appears that we are willing to accept some very high risks voluntarily (driving) but only very small involuntary risks (toxic waste). For example, we choose between the vicissitudes of nature on an unprotected flood plain and the potentially more catastrophic hazard associated with dams and levees. Kates, interviewing flood victims, found that many believed the incident could not ever happen again, while others believed that new dams would prevent the problem in the future (22). Others attempt to reduce the risk by outlawing it.

The real problem in many cases is improved technology. For example, better highways may decrease the death toll per vehicle mile driven but better highways may also increase the total number of deaths because more miles are driven. Thus, efforts to eliminate a risk may only change its form. Cohen explained thatthe most serious risk you run in the United States is remaining unmarried. A much more recognised risk, of course, is cigarette smoking. While overweight and disease are also serious risks, Cohen found that probably the least recognised major risk was more a socio-economic one, being poor, unskilled, and under-educated. Cohen demonstrated that 'dropping out of school at an early age ranks with taking up smoking as one of the most dangerous acts a young person can perform' (23).

It is also obvious that there is an extremely wide gap in perception of risk between the lay person and the supposed expert. Three good examples of what can happen can be seen in the United States with the saccharin, cyclamate, and nitrite decisions made by the Food and Drug Administrationa and, after public pressure, also our Congress. The American public asked why can't you experts make a reasonable, rational, judgement? Many lay people believed that the decisions were easy and simple. Only we, the experts, had problems. They were right. We were bogged down in data and found a different answer from almost every expert. The lay people only had summary information from the press and media. Thus, they saw the issues in black and white, a simple 'yes' or 'no'. Perhaps they saw things more clearly.

The public, at least in the United States, has grown distrustful of the expert which explains the bumper sticker on some automobiles that reads, 'Caution; Life is Hazardous to your Health'. We scientists keep talking more technically and more and more to ourselves. This further frustrates and alienates the lay people because they feel they are dealing with paternalistic scientists, who will take care of them. We imply, or even state, that they should not worry because we experts will make the right decision for you. Callahan has discussed four issues that need attention in this area of paternalism. They are (1) mystification (retreating into technical jargon when one's expertise is questioned), (2) failure to make clear the limitations of the technique being used (limitations of technique should be very precise and one should not be left in doubt on what the limitations are and what that means to the decision being made), (3) failure to distinguish facts from values (concept of risk, an empirical concept, is different from the concept of safety, a normative concept), and (4) making clear one's own value premise (choice of methodology can be based on one's own values - is there such a thing as value-free science or value-free technique or methodology) (24).

The determination of an acceptable level of risk for society cannot be made solely by the scientist or the regulator because that leaves out a considerable number of the people whom the decision affects. Thus, the social and behavioural sciences must be brought into the equation. Slovic et al have studied the answers of ordinary lay people to the question of how safe is safe enough? They found that perceived risk is quantifiable and predictable, that it means different things to different people and that, even when groups disagree about the overall risk of specific hazards, they show remarkable agreement when rating these hazards or characteristics of risk (25,26).

O'Riordan summarises the present problem as: 'The loss of faith among certain groups in modern Western society with the honesty and competence of those who assess and finally make judgements about public safety. The problem lies as much in a suspicion over the motives of leading personalities and the fidelity of assessment procedures as it does with the collective psychology of individual beliefs and judgements' (27). In the United States, there is a societal policy that the public must be informed and involved in the decision-making. Education of the public and disclosure of all the facts is terribly important from not only an ethical standpoint, but from an educational standpoint, so that the most informative, but not necessarily the most technically correct, answer can be garnered.

What can risk assessment do? Currently, risk assessment is a fairly controversial subject for many of the reasons already stated. However, risk assessment can be used to rank risks and thus set priorities. It can be used to obtain quantitative information and, in the case of chemicals, it can be used to determine action levels.

What further needs to be done? First, we must develop better technical data. At present, the technical aspects are fraught with uncertainty and too many assumptions. When we attempt to estimate risk precisely, lay people believe that these numbers are precise just like a pH meter giving the pH of a solution. Instead, our numbers are, at best, like pH paper readings. Therefore, we must develop better quality in our data. Second, we must find better ways to approach the question of what the public considers to be an acceptable risk. Third, we must develop a method for comparing risks, so that the public will begin to understand the nature of a new risk based on the risks they are already accepting. I call this the risk-assessment ladder. Certain risks (poisoning of the food supply) we will never accept. Other risks we will have to decide on based on a multi-disciplinary team of qualified scientists, regulators, and the lay public. I believe it is only in this manner that we can get all those affected by the decision involved in the decision-making process.

References
1. Giovacchini, R P. Old and new issues in the safety evaluation of cosmetics and toiletries. CRC Critical Review in Toxicology, 1, 361-378, 1972.
2. Wilson, R. Proposed regulations for identification, clarification, and regulation of toxic substances posing a potential occupational carcinogenic risk. Direct Testimony, Occupational Safety and Health, US Congress Docket No H-090, 1978.
3. Pott, P. Chirurgical observations relative to the cataract, the polypus of the nose, the cancer of the scrotum, the different kinds of rupture, and the mortification of the toes and the feet. L Hawes, W Clarke and R Collins, p 63, London, 1775.
4. Lowrance, W W. Of acceptable risk. William Kaufman Inc, Los Altos, California, 1976.
5. Otway, H J. Risk estimations and evaluations. Proc of IIASA Planning Conference on Energy Systems. International Institute for Applied Systems Analysis, Lehoss, Laxenburg, Austria, 1973.
6. Wodicka, V O et al. Proposed system for food safety assessment. Scientific Committee, Food Safety Council, Fd Drug and Cosmet Toxicol, *16*, Suppl. 2, 1978.
7. Rodricks, J V. Scientific basis for identifying potential carcinogens and estimating their risks. Interagency Regulatory Liason Group (IRLG) Room 500, Washington DC, 1979.
8. Crump, K S. Theoretical problems in the modified Mantel-Bryan procedure. Biometrics, *33*, 752-775, 1977.
9. Hartley, H O and Seilken, R L. Estimation of 'safe doses' in carcinogenic experiments. Biometrics, *33*, 1-10, 1977.

10. Brown, C C. Statistic aspects of extrapolation of dichotomous dose-response data. JNCI, *60*, 101-108, 1978.
11. Carlborg, F W. Multi-stage dose response models in carcinogenesis. Fd Cosmet Toxicol, *19*, 361-365, 1981.
12. Anderson, M W et al. A general scheme for the incorporation of pharmacokinetics in low-dose risk estimation for chemical carcinogenesis: example, vinyl chloride. Toxicol Appl Pharmacol, *55*, 154-161, 1980.
13. Iverson, S and Arley, H. On the mechanism of experimental carcinogenesis. Acta Path Microbial Scand, 27, 773-803, 1950.
14. Rai, K and Von Ryzin, J. A generalized multi-hit dose-response model for low-dose extrapolation. Biometrics, *37*, 341,352, 1981.
15. Haseman, J K et al. Some practical problems arising from use of the gamma multi-hit model for risk estimation. J Toxicol Environ Health, *8*, 379-386, 1981.
16. Druckrey, H. Quantitative aspects in chemical carcinogenesis. UICC Monograph Series, Potential Carcinogenic Hazards from Drugs, 7, 60-78, Springer-Verlag, New York, 1967.
17. Jones, H B and Grendon, A. Environmental factors in the origin of cancer and estimation of the possible hazard to man. Fd Cosmetic Toxicol, *13*, 251-268, 1975.
18. Pike, M C. A method of analysis of a certain class of experiments in carcinogenesis. Biometrics, *22*, 142-162, 1966.
19. Scheuplein, R. Risk assessment of 2,4-DAA in hair dyes, NDELA in cosmetics and saccharin in foods. Memo to Albert C Kolbye Jr et al, Department of Health Education and Welfare, Public Health Service, Food and Drug Administration, March 27, 1978.
20. USDA/FDA Announcement on Nitrites and Related Issues. Hearing before the Committee on Agriculture, House of Representatives, Ninety-Sixth Congress, Second Session, Serial No 96-VVV, 2-110, September 16, 1980.
21. Hutt, P. Public participation in toxicology decisions. Symposium: Toxicology in Transition, Toronto, Canada, 1977.
22. Kates, R W. Hazard and choice perception in flood plain management. Research Paper 78, Department of Geography, University of Chicago, Illinois, 1962.
23. Cohen, B L. The risks you run. Consumer Research Magazine, 16-20, May, 1981.
24. Callahan, D. Decisions in the real world: regulatory implications. Ethical uses of risk/benefit analyses. Symposium on risk/benefit decisions and the public health. Proceedings of the Third FDA Science Symposium, February 15-17, 1958, pp 71-74. Ed: J A Staffa, FDA, Rockville, Maryland.
25. Slovic, P et al. Rating the risks. Environment, *21*, 14-20, 36-39, 1979.
26. Slovic, P et al. Why study risk perception? Risk Analysis, *2*, 83-89, 1982.
27. O'Riordan, T. Risk-perception studies and policy priorities. Risk Analysis, *2*, 95-100, 1982.

11
The empirical approach: vinyl chloride - a cancer case study

I F CARNEY

Vinyl chloride monomer (VCM) is a simple organic chemical gas which is normally handled in industry as a pressurised liquid. It was discovered about 1833 and 5 years later its polymerisation was observed. Its main use now is in the manufacture of PVC (polyvinyl chloride) and for this purpose around 12 million tonnes are produced annually throughout the world.

The first evidence of worker health problems with VCM appeared in the early 1960s. Men who entered the PVC autoclaves and were thus exposed to high concentrations of VCM developed acro-osteolysis and as a result of animal studies to investigate this condition, carcinogenic properties were also suspected. Beginning April 1973, Maltoni was reporting the rare tumour, angiosarcoma of the liver (ASL) from his rat experiments. One year later the first human ASL cases were recorded in the USA. These events prompted intense activity throughout the world because a chemical of evident economic importance was recognised as a human carcinogen. The immediate response was a planned reduction in worker exposure to VCM from a previous 200 ppm (TLV) to less than 5 ppm, though shortly before that the TLV had been 500 ppm.

There have now been nearly 1000 articles published in the scientific press on all aspects of VCM toxicity and its relevance to man. If such publications are considered with the many on quantitative risk assessment there are a very large number of answers offered to the all-important question,'what is a safe concentration of VCM for human exposure?' In fact, the question needs refining to be meaningful and it has most frequently become 'what is the most precise and accurate estimate of the concentration of VCM in air which increases the lifetime risk of ASL in exposed humans by 1 in 1 000 000?'

There are two main sources of data for such estimates (i) studies in experimental animals and (ii) analysis of effects in humans - or epidemiological studies.

Studies in experimental animals
In terms of quantitative risk estimates, the chronic animal bioassay has provided most data. Such studies give information on the numbers of animals in different dose groups which exhibit cancer and permit the application of mathematical techniques most favoured by the investigator.

Table 1. *Lowest concentrations of VCM giving significant excess of tumours in rats (Maltoni et al 1981)*

Stomach (papilloma)	30 000 ppm
Zymbal gland	10 000 ppm
Nephroblastoma	250 ppm - female
	100 ppm - male
Liver angiosarcoma	200 ppm - male
	50 ppm - female
Mammary gland	5 ppm - female

Maltoni and co-workers have made the largest contribution with their 17 studies on VCM (1). Carcinogenic effects were observed in mice, rats and hamsters although unavoidable biological variation and changes in procedure complicate the interpretation of these, as many other animal studies (see Table 1).

Barr has compiled a summary table of Maltoni's five main experiments in rats which developed ASL. Four of the five experiments were conducted

Table 2. *ASL incidence (%) in rats*

		Experiment number:			
	1	2	7*	9	15
Dose (ppm)					
10 000	12		27		
6000	22		6.6		
2500	10		10		
500	5		13		
250			3.3		
200		10			
150		5			
100		0.8			
50	1.7		0	4.8	
25					4.2
10					0.8
5					0
1					0

* Wistar strain rats

with Sprague-Dawley strain rats, but one with Wistar strain. The difficulties of analysing such data to determine the highest, non-carcinogenic dose of VCM to rats can be appreciated from Table 2.

One important feature of making animal data meaningful to man is to check for the similarity of metabolic pathways for VCM in both species. For the rat it is now accepted that highly reactive intermediates in the metabolic process (particularly chlorethylene oxide and chloracetaldehyde) react with cellular macro-molecules, including DNA producing the critical lesions leading to mutation or the induction of cancer. From obviously limited studies using human liver tissue this proposed pathway and end-result is believed to be similar in rodents and man.

However, another feature is equally important for extrapolation from animals to man and that is reaction kinetics or whether the end-result is the same irrespective of the dose given; such information is crucial in the risk assessment for VCM. Gehring et al (2) discovered that as the dose of VCM administered to rats was increased then a smaller proportion of the dose was actually converted, or metabolised in comparison to the proportion converted from a low dose and thus kinetics were non-linear at higher concentrations. It was later found that an equilibrium is quickly established between VCM concentrations in the blood and atomosphere and that there was little or no storage of VCM in the body. Therefore factors for accumulation would not have to be incorporated into calculations of risk.

In summary therefore, animal studies have established: a link between VCM and experimental ASL; that the relationship is dose dependent; that the metabolites of VCM are probably responsible for ASL in the rat and man; and that extrapolation from low doses is, at best, uncertain.

Data from human exposure
Manufacture and use of VCM and PVC could result in potential exposure of 4 groups of the population :
(1) The highest exposure category are the workers involved in the manufacture of VCM and its polymerisation to PVC. In this group certain occupations such as autoclave cleaning would have had higher potential exposure than others (although all groups would now be expected to have exposures below 1 to 3 ppm hygiene standards). The evidence suggests that in the past some autoclave workers may have been exposed to extremely high levels of VCM.

(2) Workers in the compounding and fabrication of PVC products would have been exposed to levels 10 to 100 times lower than those in group 1. In a study of 4341 deaths from 17 PVC factories in the USA, no cases of ASL or any excess of lung or brain cancers were found, any evidence that intestinal and urinary cancers were increased in incidence has not been confirmed. In the UK, very similar results were obtained in a study of 707 deaths of male fabrication workers.

(3) Consumers who eat food and drink beverages which have been packed in PVC may ingest unreacted VCM which has migrated from the package. Since 1974 stringent controls have ensured that average daily intakes of VCM in food and drink are lower than 1 microgram/kg/day. (In a severe life-time study, Feron et al (3) induced ASL in rats by ensuring there was absorption from the stomach for 24 hr/day. The minimum dose leading to ASL was 5000 times the 1 microgram/kg/day limit.)

(4) This group would be those who live in the vicinity of VCM or PVC plants. The levels in ambient air around a factory are very low (in the parts per billion of air) but of course, large populations of all age and health groups are involved. At least 10 major studies have been made of the general population using ASL as the marker, but none of these has shown a connection between general ambient exposure and increased incidence of cancer (4).

For risk assessment purposes therefore the relationship between ASL and VCM must be examined in group 1. ASL is a rare - but not unknown - cancer in unexposed populations so its presence in VCM/PVC workers can reasonably be attributed to VCM exposure. The data-base for this purpose is the ASL Register; from 1974 cases from around the world have been recorded and categorised. The register is now maintained by Dr John Stafford of Imperial Chemical Industries who has updated and circulated it to interested parties in Universities, Governments, Trade Unions and research organisations etc. At the end of 1982, 99 cases had been included and following analyses by country, company and plant etc, some important conclusions emerge:

* The majority of ASL cases are PVC autoclave cleaners or men who worked in or around the autoclaves.

* ASL tends to occur in larger numbers in some plants than in others, 87% of USA cases originate from just 4 plants, whereas 40 plants have not so far recorded one case.

* The average latent period between starting work in an occupation with VCM exposure and death from ASL for the 99 cases is 21.9 years.

* All 99 cases were first exposed before the mid 1960s which coincides with discovery of acro-osteolysis and improved procedures for autoclave cleaning.

Therefore we have as yet no information about whether these improvementshave had any effect on the incidence of ASL in exposed populations.

Risk assessment from animal and human data

Maltoni's experiments have been the basis for many estimates of a 10^{-6} lifetime risk to man which cover a substantial range (up to 10^8), depending on the mathematical model and the inherent assumptions. Even after more 'selective' estimates have been derived - for instance, by correcting for the non-linear kinetics of metabolism at high doses - a large range of 10^3 in 'low risk dose estimate' is obtained. Clearly at this stage in their development we can have little confidence in mathematical models for quantitative risk estimates from animal studies. At a joint NIOSH and OSHA conference in 1980 to 'Re-evaluate the Toxicity of Vinyl Chloride and PVC' the conclusion was reached that no reliable estimate of human risk can be obtained from raw animal data alone, but it must include biological adjustments.

Turning to the human data therefore, about 19 epidemiological studies of cancer associated with VCM have been undertaken since 1974. Several have been criticised, but when considered alongside the animal data to estimate the exposure for 1 in 1 000 000 life-time risk, some 15 different values have emerged. The estimates have ranged from 0.000 000 39 to 1400.0 parts per billion depending on, amongst other things, which theory of cancer response is chosen (eg probit, logit, Weibull, one-hit, multi-hit etc.)

Accordingly, it seems that empirical, quantitative risk assessments have contributed little definitive guidance. It is certainly reasonable to suggest that the present VCM hygiene levels of 1 to 3 ppm applied in most industrialised countries represent an achievable best practice rather than the outcome of an acceptable and clearly defined risk assessment. The Gehring/Anderson estimate - generally regarded asthe most meaningful - of 1 ppm for 10-**6** lifetime risk was not proposed until 1980, wellafter the 1 to 3 ppm standards had been common industrial practice. Yet these conclusions are not to imply the irrelevance of empirical risk analysis for VCM, rather they illustrate that there is still very much to learn about the analyses and their application. For instance, almost all cases of ASL are associated with VCM exposure but relatively few of those exposed have developed ASL and this applies as much to rats as humans. The models leave this observation unexplained although it is clearly important in risk estimation.

The empirical information is available - the theory must be developed so that the true risk can be presented for judgement.

Acknowledgements
I wish to record my thanks to Drs Purchase, Paddle and Stafford of Imperial Chemical Industries PLC for their help in preparing this presentation.

References
1. Maltoni C et al. Environ Health Perspectives, *41*, 3-29, 1981.
2. Gehring P J et al. Tox Appl Pharmacol *44*, 581-591, 1978.
3. Feron V J et al. Fd Cosmet Toxicol, *19*, 317-333, 1981.
4. Barr J T. Hazard evaluation and risk assessment for vinyl chloride. Prepared for AICH Risk Assessment Sub-committee. March 1982.

12
Biological considerations

JENS S SCHOU

Risk is a compound phenomenon. To estimate risk a number of biological processes has to be taken into account - from the exposure of man to a certain chemical, through the possible toxicity elicited by interaction with macro-molecules in the organism and ending by final transformation to inactive metabolites.

Each link in this process has to be analysed from qualitative and quantitative points of view when risk is being estimated, and this is of course necessary if we are to discuss the acceptability of a certain level of risk. It is important to realize that risk exists and cannot be avoided completely and that reactions are very diverse reaching from slight irritative effects to the provocation of malignancies or defects of coming generations.

The difference, however, between acute effects and effects after long-term exposure or delayed onset is that the acute effects are recognized in connection with a recognizable exposure, while the late occuring effects often result from an unrecognized exposure often of low quantity, but during a prolonged exposure period. When a certain chemical can provoke both different acute effects, and the exposure further may lead to long term effects, the long term effects usually have to be considered the dominating risk when estimating the maximum tolerable level of exposure. This is due to the fact that they usually occur after significantly lower exposure levels than those leading to acute effects. Therefore, the estimation of acute toxicity of a carcinogen in general can be considered as nonsense.

Routes of exposure
The exposure of man to a chemical is either through the skin, through the respiratory system or the alimentary canal. The route of the exposure is of relevance for the character and quantity of the chemical interaction with the organism, as the metabolism and the binding processes and thereby the pharmacokinetics for organic molecules may differ depending on the exposure route. Both the quantity and quality of metablic processes show differences, as shown by an example with a drug like dextropropoxiphene. In this case a very significant first-pass metabolism after oral intake leads to high concentrations of the potentialy toxic metabolite desmethylpropoxiphene or norpropoxiphene, while the metabolite is almost undetectable after parenteral exposure. This also means that the risk of toxicity of the same amount of the molecule is very different with oral and parenteral exposure.

There are several factors which lead to differences in response depending on the route of exposure. The skin and the mucous membranes in the respiratory and alimentary tract all show different penetration qualities and they also react differently to physical and chemical stimuli. The skin normally forms a reasonable barrier against uptake of foreign components, especially in gas form. However, organic solvents may be taken up as highly lipid soluble materials, such as organophosphates. The organic solvents on the skin may add to the amount taken up from inhaling vapours, eg when house painters are cleaning their hands with mineral turpentine.

On the other hand the alveolar membrane is a very delicate structure with low resistance to penetration by foreign material which in gas form reaches the absorptive part of the lung. The lung is without the protective apparatus formed by the enzymes in the gastro-intestinal system. While the alimentary canal has a chemical protection system, the airways only present a physical hindrance for particles over a certain size (about 1 micron depending on the geometry and the specific weight) to reach the alveolar space.

Local phenomena

When the skin, an external or an internal mucous membrane is exposed to a foreign molecule three things may be the result: it may either be expelled without any interaction with the surface, or a chemical reaction with the tissues can lead to either reversible or irreversible changes. The reversible reactions are mainly of vascular character, often elicited through the liberation of local hormones, such as histamine or 5-hydroxytryptamine. The symptoms are erthyema and swelling, transitory phenomena which disappear when the chemical irritant is removed from the site of reaction.

Irreversible reactions may result from corrosive effects of strong acids or bases or from action of chemicals leading to cellular damage and to destruction of tissues by other mechanisms of cytotoxicity. Cytotoxicity to somatic cells, however, does not always lead to cellular death, as oncogenesis may result in tumour formation. Well-known examples are asbestosis which in man involves diffuse interstitial fibrosis in the lung, pleural calcification and fibrosis, bronchogenic carcinomas and mesothelial tumours. The occurence of nasopharyngeal tumours in rats exposed to formaldehyde is well established, although the consequences for man are difficult to determine. This is also an example of the dilemma concerning species differences in the extrapolation from animal experiments to risk in man.

Absorptive effects

After absorption, most xenobiotics (foreign chemicals or 'guest molecules') in the organism interact with the host organism in one way or another. This may both affect the guest molecules as well as the host organism, the foreign micro-molecule interacting with macro-molecules of the organism. However, some chemical entities are inert and leave the organism unchanged either through the lungs as narcotic gases or through the urine. This on the other hand does not mean that the organism is unaffected during their passage, as can be seen with the effects of narcotic gases.

The foreign molecules may interact either with extra-cellular systems as when they bind to albumin or other protein systems, with biological membranes, or they penetrate into cells to affect intra-cellular structures or to be affected by intra-cellular enzyme systems. Binding to cell membranes may change the condition of the cell by altering the cell membrane potential or the permeability and thereby causing insufficient energy supply to maintain the optimal function of the cell.

The parenchymal cells of the liver are easily penetrated by most foreign molecules and their enzyme systems are suitable for the transformation of organic molecules. This is not the place for a further description of synthetic and non-synthetic biotrans formation of foreign molecules. It should be emphasised, however, that the P-450 system and other enzymes do not always lead to formation of biologically inert or less reactive molecules than the original xenobiotic.

It is well-known that intermediary products in metabolic chain reactions may be of high reactivity with macro-molecules of vital importance. An example is the formation of epoxides (Figure) which may bind covalently to DNA and thereby in

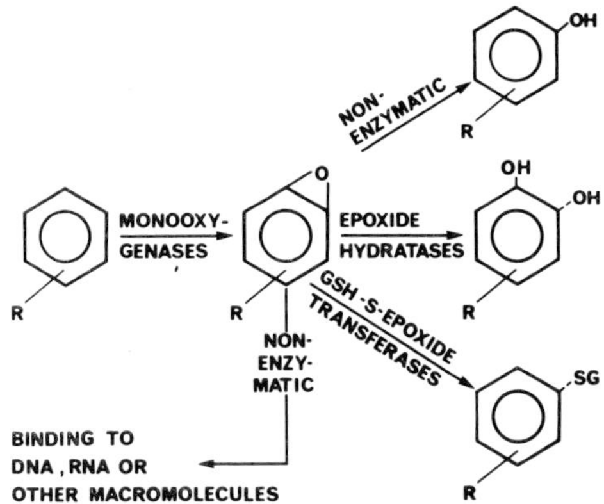

Figure.
*A model presentation showing a xenobiotic molecule being transformed into a highly reactive epoxide metabolite.*This is a transitory molecule being transformed into inactive metabolites mainly by glutathione-S-epoxide transferase. The capacity of this enzyme is limited and may be saturated, leading to toxicity by accumulating amounts of the epoxide binding to DNA and RNA or other macro-molecules.

certain cases lead to changes in cell reproduction and cell properties. In the reaction pattern shown, low amounts of the foreign molecule lead to formation of epoxides at a rate which is easily followed by the inactivation processes. The latter may be rate limited, however, and if high amounts of the foreign chemical are administered they can be saturated, and a free surplus of epoxide results and may cause trouble.

Special reactivity
The description of the epoxide problems which occur when the inactivating systems are saturated implies that a clear dose-effect relationship does not necessarily exist for toxic reactions. This is also the case with long-term effects or delayed effects, where 'dose' has to be considered a function of the level of exposure and the duration of exposure. Often the exposure period is interrupted by exposure-free intervals and the magnitude of exposure varies during the exposure periods. Other reactions occurring without a clear-cut dose relationship are intolerance reactions and allergies following sensitisation to chemicals.

It should not be forgotten that a significant health problem is associated with allergy and intolerance reactions to man-made chemicals in terms of severity of the clinical condition, seriousness of interference with life quality and in the large number of exposed people. Only epidemiological investigations can elucidate the occurrence of skin and respiratory tract hyper-sensitivity and only limited data are available.

There is a lack of predictive tests in humans with regard to antibody-mediated hypersensitivities of the respiratory tract and the skin. With respect to the dose-effect problem, it shoud be noted that the exposure levels and lengths of exposure to initiate antibody formation are, in general, higher than those necessary for eliciting later clinical manifestations. In summary, it is not clearly known whether a dose-effect relationship exists in chemically induced allergic phenomena. This is an area of research which should be given high priority due to the great number of people affected by such reactions.

Special risk groups
When animal experiments are performed for safety assessment, young adult male rats
are the most commonly used experimental animal. But young adult men represent
only a limited part of the population which is exposed to any kind of potentially
dangerous chemicals. We have in any safety evaluation to take into account the part of
the population with the highest sensitivity to the hazardous effects of the new
compounds. We therefore have to pay special attention to the very young and the very
old, to the pregnant woman and her progeny and to patients with decreased resistance
due to disease processes.

It should be remembered that the foetus, due to haemodynamic conditions,
is especially exposed to high concentrations of un-metabolised xenobiotics taken up
by the pulmonary route. Similar conditions exist for the central nervous system. The
reason is that by pulmonary uptake the absorbed material passes with the pulmonary
venous blood directly to the left side of the heart and is therefore pumped directly and
undiluted to the brain and the foetus.

On the other hand, when materials are taken up though the skin the venous
blood through the right side of the heart is pumped through the lung circulation,
including the capillary bed before coming to the arterial system through the left side of
the heart. When xenobiotics are taken up from the alimentary canal, not only the lung
(as described for the skin uptake), but also the liver with its high metabolic capacity is
inserted as a 'filter'. This means that before the xenobiotic reaches the arterial blood it
has been through one or two filters and the venous blood from the site of uptake has
been diluted by mixing with the venous blood from the rest of the body. Only after
pulmonary uptake is there a much more direct exposure of the tissues to the amount
absorbed. Therefore also haemodynamic factors and special sensitivity groups have
to be included in safety assessment.

Can risk be defined in biological terms?
What has been said until now can in a way be considered as a prelude to the main
question: does there exist an acceptable risk from a biological point of view? By
definition risk is the possibility or likelihood of danger or injury, meaning that it is a
statistical phenomenon.

I feel convinced that the biologist cannot help establishing limits to acceptable
risk. The biologist can describe the processes leading to injury or hazards. We can
describe the complexity of events leading from exposure to injury and we can quantify
the phenomena by dose-effect relationships. We can help by extrapolating from
dose-effect phenomena in animal experiments to possible dose relationships in man
and we can list all the factors that under all conditions make it uncertain to conclude
from one species to another. We can from experience conclude that, with respect to
carcinogenicity testing, the only definite conclusion to be drawn from a positive or
negative experiment on rats is that the substance investigated in the species used and
under the given conditions does or does not increase the occurrence of malignancies.
We know too many examples today of species-specific tumours and of hormonal
reactivity in malignancies which are species-specific, too.

It is therefore my personal opinion today that we get close to the point where
a relevant test battery of short-term tests gives answers to the question of human
carcinogenicity with the same degree of truth as the long-term animal experiments.
However, the short-term tests have to be selected carefully, they have to include tests
on mammalian cells and on intact animals, and they have to be well validated. But I
hope that we can soon get away from the time consuming and extremely expensive
long-term experiments.

The biologist may help to select the major hazard problems when one component may lead to a number of different injuries. We also know that life itself has a natural risk which, for each step in life, can be calculated statistically; but also here is a magnitude of confounding factors, such as ethnic factors, environmental factors, hygiene and so on. Also the product areas have to be taken into account when trying to decide which level of risk is to be accepted; and as acceptance has to be decided from a social point of view, it is a decision to be taken by politicians who weigh up the different hazards against each other.

When a biologist considers the problem of 'the acceptable risk', we reach the conclusion that we can describe the mechanisms and complexity of risk, we know that we cannot exist without risk, but the decision of the acceptable risk has to be balanced against the social need or wish for the use of the chemical or product. The same attitude has to be taken when the problem is raised whether carcinogens are acceptable in our surroundings and in products for human use if they can be shown not to interact with essential tissues. But nor to this question is there a sound biological answer.

13
Perceived risk: a chimera?

JACK DOWIE

The main risk in attending conferences is that the speaker is not very good at diagnosing the condition of knowledge deficiency in advance. He may lack *sensitivity* - have a high false negative rate - and *frustrate* you to death by not telling you what you want to be told. Or he may lack specificity - have a high false positive rate - and *bore* you to death by telling you what you don't need to be told. I hope I can at least achieve an acceptable balance between boredom and frustration.

It's almost obligatory to begin talks about perception with two pictures. Showing the first, vase/faces or 'figure'/'ground', picture (Figure 1) is sometimes designed, I suspect, to upset the audience, suggesting to them (by analogy) that what they *hear* is only one of at least two valid interpretations of what is being said. Listened to in one way we hear a benign vase (eg a well balanced rational treatment), listened to in another way we hear two hostile faces (eg an emotional polemic). Of course we all agree, don't we, that there *is* no objectively correct *single* thing to see. Whether the vase is the 'figure' and the faces the 'ground' or vice versa *does* depend on *how* we see, not on what is *there*: being sophisticated we know that there *are* two things there to be seen, each of which has equal potential to become 'figure' or 'ground'.

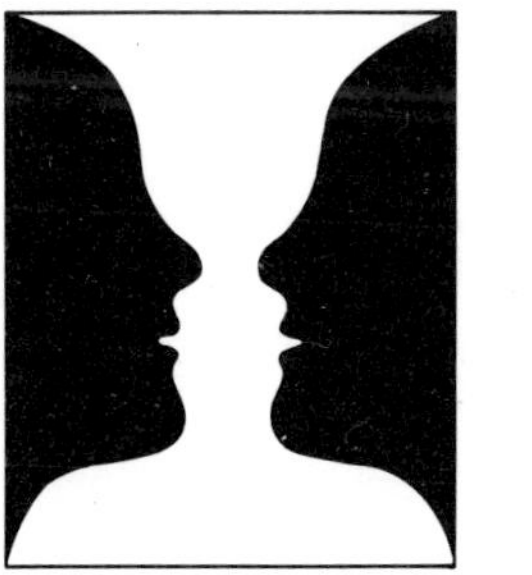

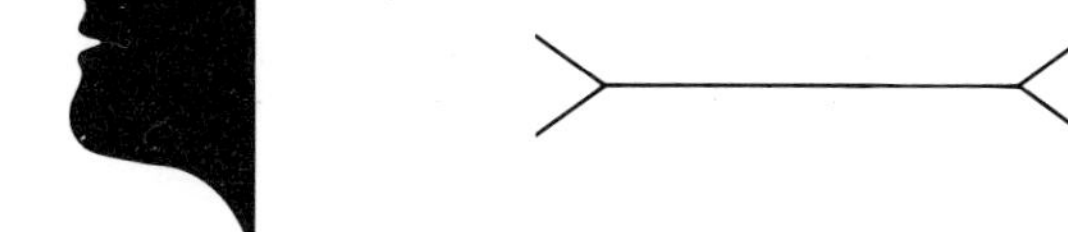

Figure 1   Figure 2

Things are a bit different with the arrowed lines (Figure 2) (the Muller-Lyer illusion). When the unsophisticated assert that the lower horizontal line is longer, our self satisfaction arises from knowing that there *is* an objectively correct answer: the lines are actually equal in length.

Much of the debate about risk perception over the last decade seems to me to have been a debate about which of these is the appropriate analogy. Those who favour the 'lines' analogy devise what they see as the single objective measure of the risk in an activity, ask individuals for their assessments of the risk in it, say 'spot the difference!', and characterise that difference as misperception or bias. Whether the arrowheads that produce the bias are supplied by the perceiver, trying to see what he wants to see, or appear before his eyes through some unmotivated process, becomes the only issue. (Both possibilities are of course compatible with highly motivated *efforts* by *others* - advertisers, politicians, pressure groups - to create arrowheads of particular shapes and sizes.) (Should I add educators?) At the other extreme those who favour the 'faces/vase' analogy argue that there are totally legitimate alternative character-isations of the risk in an activity and that it will be our individual and cultural mind set that determines whether we see a benign vase or hostile faces. (In the case of nuclear power, for example, whether we see a mushroom-shaped cloud or a mushroom-lightbulb - Figure 3.) Of course the implication is that there are always just *two* possible characterisations, rather that there will be more than one, often many. My own inclination is, you will soon discern, towards the vase and faces school, though with a modification that may make 'lines' people not entirely unhappy. (The middle ground is always attractive. The only question is whether it constitutes a tenable

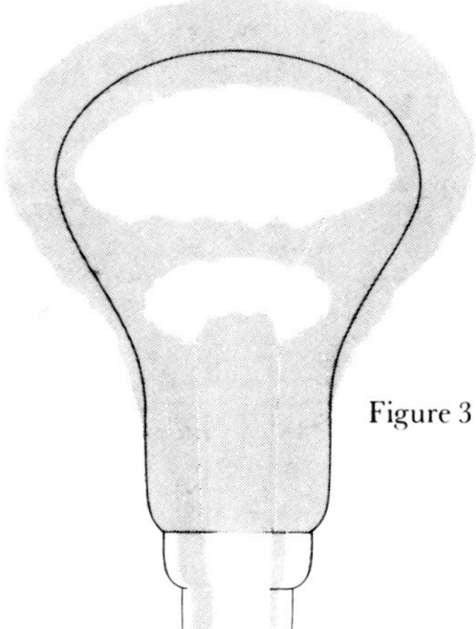

Figure 3

position logically, psychologically and sociologically.)

I fear I sound like a social scientist. Three of the most eminent researchers into risk - Paul Slovic, Sarah Lichtenstein and Baruch Fischhoff of Decision Research, Oregon - have enunciated what I shall call the Eugene 'no-win' dilemma:

> If social scientists describe their work in technical jargon no one wants to listen.
> If they use plain language, no one feels a need to listen (1).

I'm going to try to avoid the dilemma by talking Greek. Perceived risk is a chimera.

The original chimera was one of those fabulous monsters that populate the Greek myths - in the days when, since Clint Eastwood didn't exist to ride out and impose order on chaos, it was necessary to invent him.

Once upon a time there was a young Prince, called Bellerophon, grandson of Sisyphus of rolling stone fame. Bellerophon had to leave town rather hurriedly after killing two men, including his brother. King Proteus took him in, to the delight of the Queen. But Bellerophon unwisely rejected the advances of the wife of his host and she sought revenge by telling her husband that Bellerophon had made advances to her. Unable to breach the rules of hospitality Proteus asked his wife's father to kill

Bellerophon on his behalf. Father accordingly invited him to go on what he thought would be a suicide mission against the chimera, a beast which had been giving the area lots of trouble and despatching the best soldierssent against it. Its fire-breathing lion's head was joined to the agile body of a mountain goat; it had a venemous serpent for a tail.

Bellerophon consulted that early form of risk assessor called a soothsayer, who told him that he would only be able to slay the chimera if he was mounted on the winged horse Pegasus. With the help of a golden bridle given him by the Goddess Athene, Bellerophon captured Pegasus and set out to attack the monster. Dodging the flames, he fired arrow after arrow, which crippled it. Then, to finish it off he fixed a large lump of lead to the end of his spear and thrust it down into the fiery mouth. The lead melted and streamed down into the chimera's stomach, with fatal consequences.

Bellerophon returned triumphant, but only after many other dangerous tasks had been accomplished did father realise his daughter must have been fibbing. The truth finally emerged and, believe it or not, Bellerophon was given the hand of the Queen's younger sister as compensation.

Unfortunately, they didn't live happily ever after. Bellerophon became insufferably conceited about his exploits, compared himself with the Gods and decided he would visit them on Olympus, using Pegasus. An outraged Zeus sent a gadfly to sting Pegasus in mid-air, he reared and unseated his rider, who fell to earth, where he wandered around, crippled and alone, until he eventually died.

The moral? That comes at the end.

The myth updated

Each and every human activity gives birth to and sustains a chimera, so they come in vast variety and number. How many varieties and what numbers are major sources of disagreement among professional chimera-watchers, as well as the ordinary person getting on with daily life.

A major reason for continuing disagreement is the inability of anyone to actually capture a chimera and dissect it. The only thing which has been established beyond reasonable doubt (in my view: I have to add that) is their basic anatomy. The beasts are indeed *chimeras* - two totally different sorts of animal joined together. I am going to call one sort of animal 'a probability ' and the other sort 'an outcome'. The simplest possible chimera that can exist resides in/on a two outcome activity and may be pictured as in Figure 4a. Each outcome element (O) of a chimera is tied inseparably to a particular probability element (P).

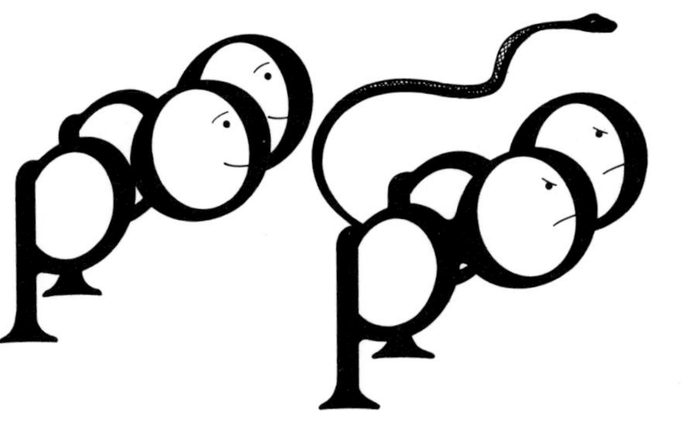

Figure 4, a and b

That's about as far as *agreement* goes (if it goes that far), but before I move to some of the disagreements, what about the serpent tail? It is my contention that the chimera only grows its tail and becomes venomous (Figure 4b) under particular conditions. By far the most important one is when we fail to see it as a chimera and treat it instead as a crossbreed, ie we lose sight of the two distinct elements that make it up and treat it as a genuine (genetic) merger, thinking that we can find out something about the beast as a whole which is not (just) the sum of what we can find out about its two components.

The second condition for 'arming' the chimera relates to the outcome half. You will be aware that there is much disagreement about how many separate outcome elements any particular chimera contains, what they are, and whether or not we can hope ever to identify all of them. Some agreement exists regarding a group of elements concerned with mortality and morbidity, though even here the room for argument is clear if I list the sort of labels that have been used:

    one instant death of a specified person
    one instant death of a random person
    twenty instant deaths in a single event
    twenty instant deaths in twenty separate incidents
    ten deaths after two years perfect health
    no deaths but two years morbidity
    lifetime disability.

When we move to other sorts of outcome element and encounter the use of (eg):

    destruction of equipment
    use of 100 units of energy
    loss of one friendship
    one year of public ridicule
    loss of '10' degrees of freedom/control,

the awesome character of the problem and the ultimately subjective/intersubjective nature of its resolution becomes patent. The second condition for 'arming' the chimera (ie envenoming it) is not however, the nitty-gritty of this outcome classification problem, but doing what I have just done - which is to study only those outcome elements which are conventionally regarded as *negatively* weighted. The chimera that lives in any human activity must have *some* positively weighted outcome elements in order to exist, so it is misleading and dangerous to try to analyse only one side of it. (It's like studying the veins but not the arteries. Or how many goals the home team scores but not how many the away team scores.)

I have only been able to spell out this second condition by introducing the concept of the *weight* of an outcome element. Even when there is complete or large agreement on how many outcome elements there are and what they are, assessment of their weight (or mass) remains. Liberals generally argue that everyone's assessment of the weight (utility) of an outcome element - or strictly the *relative* weights of outcome elements - is as 'good' as anyone else's. *My* view as to the relative disutility of 'the death of a specified individual' on the one hand and 'the deaths of ten random individuals' on the other is as valid (or invalid) as anyone else's. Others believe that they have access to *better* assessments as a result of superior moral or aesthetic sensitivity. I shan't claim this.

While almost anything goes in assessing the relative weight of the outcome elements - except that if you say outcome A is heavier than B and B than C, you should say A is heavier than C - anything does not quite go at the rear. For the third condition we must move there. The weights attached to the probability elements must add up to 100 percent for any one chimera. (This may seem trivially true but I suggest the history of civilisation would have been very different if everyone's probabilities for mutually exclusive and collectively exhaustive events had always added up to 1.0.) And the weights (percentages) should be well-calibrated: in just that proportion of cases should the associated outcome actually occur.

To summarise so far: the chimera is a necessary product of human activity and *in itself* (as distinct from the activity) is harmless - unless we overlook, ignore or deny its fundamental structure.

I take for granted that people's utility assessments differ, and while it is important and interesting to find out how they differ, there is no 'scientific' (as compared to 'moral' or 'aesthetic') basis for talking about utility assessments being better or worse in relation to each other. It is, *therefore*, pointless to talk of *risk* perceptions being more or less accurate - since risk involves value as well as uncertainty. We can't say *anything* about the chimera as a whole without saying something about each of its components.

Nothing I have said is intended to suggest that there can be anything *objective* about chimera analysis and that includes its probability half. Any measurement (weighing) of the probability of an outcome is conditional on subjective judgements concerning definitions and procedures (eg which occasions of the activity are to be regarded as identical/equivalent/exchangeable). But I would maintain that among a group of people in intersubjective agreement about these conditioning assumptions we *can* talk of probability assessments - perceptions - which are better or worse, more or less biased. (Science is the attempt to achieve such total intersubjective consensus among 'those who know most'. There is unfortunately no scientific way of defining the latter.)

The now quite extensive empirical literature on 'risk assessment' confirms to me that if we don't ask clear questions *about each half of the chimera separately* we won't get answers which can be meaningfully interpreted.

I will pick out the well-known Eugene study where clear questions were asked about the probability end and we do get a clear answer: ordinary people's assessments of mortality rates *are* systematically biased (granted that they would accept the conditioning assumptions). Slovic and his colleagues:

> ....compared the judged number of deaths per year with the actual number as reported in public health statistics. If the frequency judgements were accurate, they would equal the statistical rates, and all data points would fall on the 45 degree line. While more likely hazards generally evoked higher estimates, the points are best described as being scattered about a curved line that lies sometimes above and sometimes below the line of accurate judgement. In general, rare causes of death were overestimated and common causes of death were underestimated. As a result, while the actual death toll varied over a range of one million, average frequency judgements varied over a range of only a thousand.
>
> In addition to this general bias, many important specific biases were evident. For example, accidents were judged to cause as many deaths as diseases, whereas diseases actually take about 15 times as many lives. Homicides were incorrectly judged more frequent than diabetes and stomach cancer. Homicides were also judged to be about as frequent as a stroke, although the latter actually claims about 11 times as many lives. Frequencies of death from botulism, tornadoes and pregnancy (including childbirth and abortion) were also greatly overestimated.
>
> In keeping with the availability heuristic hypotheses, overestimated items were dramatic and sensational, whereas, underestimated items tended to be

unspectacular events, which claim one victim at a time and are common in nonfatal form (2).

Slovic et al went on to emphasize the vital role of experience as a determinant of perceived risk. 'If one's experiences are biased, one's perceptions are likely to be inaccurate. Unfortunately, much of the information to which people are exposed provides a distorted picture of the world of hazards.' As a follow-up to the studies reported above, they examined the reporting of causes of death in two newspapers on opposite coasts of the United States and found that the two were similar in their 'biased' covering of life-threatening events: the number of reports was not closely related to statistical frequencies of occurrence. All forms of disease appeared to be relatively neglected whereas violent, often catastrophic events such as tornadoes, fire, drownings, homicides, and accidents were reported disproportionately often.

Whether this media 'bias' is producer-induced ('give 'em what we want 'em to know') or consumer-induced ('give 'em what they want') is probably unresolvable, especially in the absence of a *normative* theory of news value - of what should be reported and how - to give a basis for biased measurement. As far as the latter goes it seems obvious to me that giving every individual death *equal* media coverage is a non-starter, so that a comparison of coverage and statistical frequency as officially defined can only be the basis for more complex theorising. News value, I suggest elsewhere, varies inversely with probability and directly with the absolute value of utility squared (Figure 5). Or perhaps the function is *uneven* - good news has to be proportionately much more good than bad news has to be bad to get covered. The curves are isofleets (joining all points of equal news value) and represent higher and higher news value as we move from right to left. Charles and Di marrying tomorrow is near top right, a Royal death after terminal illness has been diagnosed will be near bottom right, a social scientist going on about the real world will be halfway between

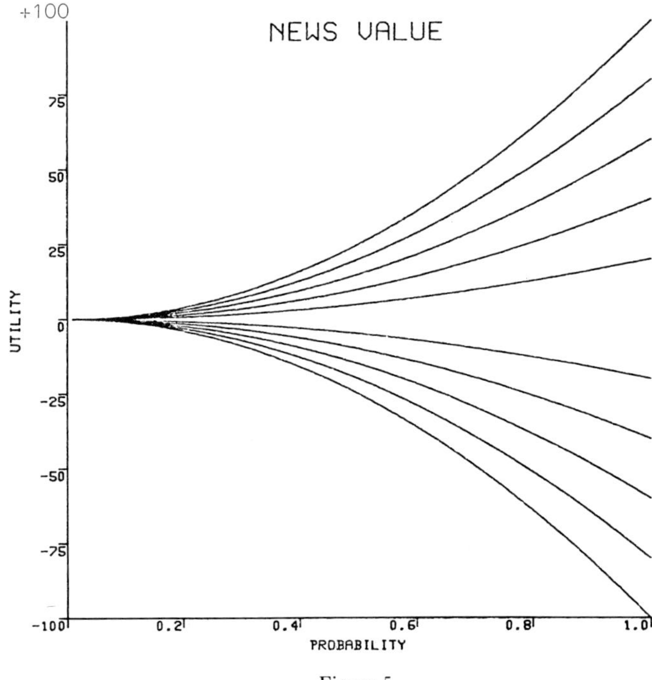

Figure 5

them on the right hand edge. You don't agree? Well of course I haven't said *whose* utilities and probabilities. All I want to do is point to the likely clash between news value and educational value and suggest that should be a priority research area in view of the role of public judgements for policy-making.

After these important pioneering studies research seems to have got diverted into pursuing the undoubtedly intriguing question of popular perceptions of the chimera *as a whole* - the chimera 'armed' by ignoring its dual nature, as well as sometimes by neglect of its positive outcome and usually by failure to establish whether the respondents' probability assessments are minimally coherent (add to 1.0). The questions asked sometimes actually framed the issues in such a way as to facilitate the 'arming'.

Instead of asking for frequency of death assessments subjects were now asked for their assessments of 'the risk of activities, as well as for ratings of the same activities on a variety of other dimensions such as 'dreadness', 'immediacy', 'familiarity', and 'controllability'. Factor analysis uncovered the underlying structure of the 'risk assessment' in terms of these other dimensions.

> ...these data suggest that risks whose severity is believed not to be controllable tend also to be seen as dread, catastrophic, hard to prevent, fatal, inequitable, threatening to future generations, not easily reduced, increasing, involuntary, and threatening to the rater personally. The nature of these characteristics suggests that this factor be called 'Dread'. The second factor primarily reflects five characteristics that correlate relatively highly with one another and less highly with other characteristics. They are: observability, knowledge, immediacy of consequences, and familiarity. We have labelled this factor 'Familiarity'. The third factor is dominated by a single characteristic, the number of people exposed (2).

What sort of questions generated the responses underlying these analyses. Here are four examples.

> Do people face this risk voluntarily?
> To what extent is the risk of death immediate?
> Is this risk new and novel or old and familiar?
> Is this a risk that people have learned to live with and can think about reasonably calmly, or is it one that people have great dread for - on the level of a gut reaction?

In each case subjects give a response on a 1-7 scale from eg 'common' to 'dread'. While I would be the last to deny that we find something out about how people think from this sort of study, it's not clear to me *what* it is or what we can do with the conclusions since we certainly don't know whether they have been armed by the chimera themselves or been talked into it by the framing of the question. *It is* important to establish (eg) whether people are less interested in the mathematical expectation than in some other characteristic of a distribution (eg its maximum possible value/catastrophic potential) but this will *not* be established by asking people 'Is this *a risk* which kills people one at a time or large numbers of people at once'.

We make progress on this question only by eliciting on the one hand their utility function in respect of number of deaths per incident and, on the other, their probabilities for incidents of varying death numbers. If we can't do that - and I don't suggest it's at all easy to do it properly - I'm unclear of the virtues of doing anything else.

I don't intend to go further into the empirical literature. I would particularly draw your attention to the important work of Brown and Green (3) in this country and Vlek and Stallen (4) in the Netherlands. To me their work raises the likelihood that ordinary people's *conception* of the chimera *may be* basically correct. Identifiable uncertainty and value dimensions keep coming through in the analyses whatever the question. Thomas and Baillie (5) point in the same direction, so that, provided *we* don't frame the questions in such a way as to distort this, we might come up with meaningful answers regarding *perceptions* of the rear end of the chimera.

Brown and Green do, incidentally, assert, on the basis of their work, that people's views of risk are highly dependent on context and specific to an activity, concluding that:

> If safety is not considered in the abstract, but only in the context of some hazard, and someone's knowledge of their preferences is dependent upon having experienced choice, then we cannot expect to achieve a simple model of preference applicable across all choices. Thus reliability can only be bought at the cost of more piecemeal models, and our desires in this field must be modest (3).

I can admire Brown and Green's humility while doubting that they see its full implications. If people do not have some abstract (I would prefer general) notion of risk and at least proto-preferences relevant to hypothetical states (death for one) - if in other words they don't see all chimeras as belonging to the same species, however different they are in their detailed anatomy - then our desires in this field need not merely be modest. They can be nil - we're surely only interested in finding out about them because we think resource allocation (defining resources in the widest possible way) can be 'improved' in some way. Fortunately, for reasons I have already given, the research, important as it is, leaves the debate still wide open.

I want to simply assert that, as far as *probability* assessments are concerned, a reasonable bet on the basis of the present research is that:

> People's assessments of *probability* are not very good, although they're far from hopeless especially when feedback is available (weather, forecasting, horse-racing).

(The issue arises as to whether many of our institutional arrangements, including laws and professional practices, are not designed to *prevent* effective feedback becoming available. *Power* might, I speculate, be defined as primarily the ability to avoid having effective feedback to one's probability assessments *generated*, secondarily, the ability to avoid the *implications* of the feedback if its generation cannot be prevented. These of course in addition to the ability to have one's *utilities* considered disproportionately highly vis-à-vis those of others.)

I'm going to spend the rest of my time noting the possible *origins* of deficiencies in probability assessments. Two major schools of thought have been in contention long before risk came to centre stage. The 'hot' contaminists locate the origins of biases in the pollution of probability judgements by what I shall call utility-end effects (emotions, drives, wishes). Freud is the biggest name, Janis and Mann (6) recent apostles.

The 'cool' contaminists locate the biases in cognitive limitations and strategies - the *unmotivated* strategies of ordinary human beings coping with information overload. Tverksy and Kahneman (7) are currently the big names.

The battle has recently been running in favour of the 'cool' school. Nisbett and Ross' *Human Inference* (8) is partly responsible. (See Sjoberg (9) for a neat short state-of-the-art assessment.) There are, however, signs that things are 'hotting up' a bit, both within cognitive psychology and in anthropology/cognitive sociology. The researchers in cognitive psychology are increasingly arguing that so-called cognitive biases have their origins in exposure to biased samples rather than biased inference from representative samples. And therefore, to the extent that exposure is *chosen*, in human action. The argument goes like this: human beings are reasonably good at assessing probabilities, *given* the experience and information they have available, they just aren't very good at realising the limitations of their experience and information and extrapolate beyond them far too readily. Coupled with a behavoural tendency to seek out a restricted range of situations (those which are populated mainly by people with the same beliefs and values) this produces the observed bias. For example I see Frank only once a fortnight at the local community aid committee and he's the epitome of the generous sociable, reasonable, altruistic chap. To his wife, who sees him in many different settings and for much longer, he is quite different. The important thing is how confidently I express (and act on) *my* judgement *outside the committee.*

As Fischoff et al (1) put it:

> One of the most robust psychological discoveries of the last 10 years has been identification of the 'fundamental attribution error', the tendency to view ourselves as highly sensitive to the demands of varying situations, but to see others as driven to consistent behaviour by dominating personality traits.... This misperception may be due to the fact that we typically see most others in only one role, as workers or spouses or parents or bowlers (ten-pin) or drivers or whatever, in which the situational pressures are quite consistent. Thus, we may observe accurately the evidence available to us, but fail to understand the universe from which these data are drawn (p 241).

That we act in such a way as to generate a biased sample of information (from which we make unbiased inferences) rather than so as to generate an unbiased sample (from which we make biased inferences) is specifically supported by the work of Snyder and colleagues on the maintenance of social stereotypes (10).

The important recent work by Mary Douglas and Aaron Wildavsky (11) advances a related argument but at the cultural (or rather subcultural) level. I can do much less than justice to their essay, but here is the gist.

There are so many human activities and hence, in my terminology so many chimeras, that we cannot possibly attend them all equally. Different social/ cultural groups, therefore, pick out different ones for priority. This selection and ordering constitutes the 'cosmology' of the group. The internal *structure* of the group (its ways of relating) must be broadly compatible with its cosmology for it to survive and function, so that one is likely to find capitalist entrepreneurs, factory workers, bureaucrats and commune dwellers emphasising the threat from different activities and rating the threat of any particular activity differently. (The leading characters in 'Dallas', 'Upstairs, Downstairs' and 'Mash', have very different chimeras in front of their mind.) This is, of course, not very exciting or novel if it is suggested to have only utility-end significance. *Of course* the (moral) values of such different groups differ and so of course, and quite legitimately, they assign different weights to the outcome elements of the same chimera. No 'hot' contamination of their probability assessments is *necessarily* involved.

But contamination is, I fear, produced by the social processes that occur in any group. It's most *obvious* (because most concentrated in space) in the communal sect but it is equally true of other groupings too. Because of its value-based interests the group spends almost all its time studying a single chimera, or small group of chimeras. Members are exposed to more and more unrepresentative samples of information, talking mainly with, and reading the work of, others who share their *values - and hence, by an unmotivated behavioural process,* their beliefs. Biased assessments of probability are not, then, individually motivated in any direct way - but they are indirectly influenced by value-motivated action. Cool and hot contamination thus occur simultaneously and interactively, so I will christen this sort of cultural bias argument the 'warm' contamination hypothesis.

This argument is, of course, simply in line with mainstream functionalist anthropology (and much common sense) in arguing that there will be close links between the attitudes of a social group and its characteristics. Mary Douglas' particular contribution (12) has been to suggest that two of these structural characteristics are sufficient to capture the main differences between types of social group *and* types of cosmology (including above all perceptions of, and attitudes to, risk). The two are (1) the degree of exclusivity and self-sufficiency of the group (how much of the activity of a member goes on within it and how firm are its boundaries with the outside world) and (2) the degree of its internal differentiation (how regulated are its members inside it in their activities and relationships). Its *groupness* and *its gridness* in her jargon.

Michael Thompson (13) has, I think, improved on this 2x2 formulation by suggesting that there is also a manipulation/power aspect and developing a model that will be familiar to catastrophe theorists. I won't go into it in detail but it does provide an intriguing explanation for such cosmological phenomena as middle-aged bureaucrats (or academics) 'dropping out' overnight to 'the good life'. The novel - and optimistic - part of his model is that it yields a *fifth* stable equilibrium cosmology/ social environment which is particularly attractive in that it seems to represent the golden mean of uncoercive coerciveness. Unfortunately (according to Thompson) only the Khumbu Sherpas of Nepal seem to have created it so far, with the help of a pretty unusual geographical situation. If this was the planners' hope for Milton Keynes I must report failure.

Much of the emphasis in Douglas and Wildavsky's work is on the inhabitants of the high group/low grid cell, which they refer to as border sects and Michael Thompson refers to as the 'survival collectivists'. For Douglas and Wildavsky they pose a serious threat to political stability in the late twentieth century, though paradoxically they can't really win. Why can't they win? Here is just a flavour of the broad argument:

> Having chosen for the sect (people) slide their decisions onto arguments that feed sectarian life; having chosen (against the sect) for the center, they slide their decisions onto center-supporting institutions. Then they are immune to reason from the other side, since center and border are structured by mutual opposition (10).
>
> The sectarian border is a kind of permanent opposition that has no intention of governing, disapproves of government, and develops no capacity for exercising power.... Since sectarian activities weaken the political center and restrict the economic room in society, the border is liable to weaken its two conditions of support....(pp 182-83).
>
> (A) harsh judgement on extreme sectarian policy only matches the notorious judgements against market competitiveness and bureaucratic stagnation. Seen in their worst light, all three forms of cultural bias are contradictory and self-defeating. Each sees particular dangers and fails to see others of its own producing.... It is easy enough to say let there be dialogue (between border and center) for a pluralistic society should work out the accommodation between initially rival and hostile views. But our analysis shows why the rival perspectives are polarized, each selecting facts to support pre-existing perceptions of risk....(p 185).

So for Douglas and Wildavsky cultural bias doesn't just produce a particular selection of risks for attention - the particular selection of risks is that bias. A (sub) culture is the risks - or chimeras - it selects for emphasis. William Clarke (14) would probably substitute 'witch' for 'chimera' and I strongly recommend his stimulating comparison of the risk hunts of the late twentieth century with the witch hunts of earlier ones.

My conclusion is, as you may have predicted, a mildly depressing one. The risk debate *has* made progress. We no longer think, as we tended to do even a few years ago, that a latter-day Bellerophon can ride out and despatch the currently fashionable chimera with a technical fix. But to assume that the implication of Douglas and Wildavsky's analysis is that the answer lies in simple 'cultural fixes' would be just as naive in its way. We have to learn to live - and die - with our chimeras because we create them in the way we live and the way we *think*. As far as the *latter* is concerned I've put in my twopenny's worth today: only when we have sorted out our conceptions (and misconceptions) of risk a lot more will we be in a good position to investigate our perceptions and misperceptions.

But, given the intimate links between the way we think and the way we relate to each other, such sorting out will not occur in a debate which lurches from this inquiry to that select committee to that Royal Commission; in which technical victory in today's match is the goal of all sides. Progress will only be made, I suggest, when mutual enlightenment is the aim of all parties, professional or lay (or anywhere between). This implies that the *debate* in fact becomes a *discourse* in which all are accorded unlimited intellectual respect and there is no set time at which one side is justified in resorting to power rather than persuasion, to ending rather than extending the conversation. I don't imply that in relation to particular current decisions one shouldn't make one's commitment and fight on the basis of one's existing beliefs and values. It is important though to be clear whether one is *equally* committed to the long haul of authentic discourse - because, if not, I offer (and accept for myself) the moral of the tale of Bellerophon. Hubris doesn't pay. In talking about most things human, perhaps risk above all, we need to be aware of how little we know - and how little we know about how much we know.

References

1. Fischhoff, B, Slovic, P and Lichtenstein, S. Lay foibles and expert fables in judgements about risk. American Statistician, *36*, 240-255, 1982.
2. Slovic, P, Fischhoff, B and Lichtenstein, S. Facts and fears: understanding perceived risk, pp 181-214. In Schwing, R C and Albers, W A (eds) Societal risk assessment: how safe is safe enough. Plenum, 1980.
3. Brown, R A and Green, C H. Threats to health or safety: perceived risk and willingness to pay. Social Science and Medicine, 15C, 67-75, 1981.
4. Vlek, C and Stallen, P J. Judging risks and benefits in the small and in the large. Organisational Behaviour and Human Performance, *28*, 235-71, 1981.
5. Thomas, K and Baillie, A. Public attitudes to the risks, costs and benefits of nuclear power. Paper prepared for a joint SERC/SSRC seminar on research into nuclear power development policies in Britain, 1982.
6. Janis, I and Mann, L. Decision making: a psychological analysis of conflict. The Free Press, 1977.
7. Tversky, A and Kahneman, D. Judgement under uncertainty: heuristics and biases. Science, *185*, 1124-31, 1974.
8. Nisbett, R and Ross, L. Human inference: strategies and shortcomings of social judgement. Prentice-Hall, 1980.
9. Sjoberg, L. Aided and unaided decision making: improving intuitive judgement. Journal of Forecasting, *1*, 349-63, 1982.
10. Snyder, M, Campbell B H and Preston, E. Testing hypotheses about human nature: assessing the accuracy of social stereotypes. Social Cognition, *1*, 256-272, 1982.
11. Douglas, M and Wildavsky, A. Risk and culture: an essay on the selection of technical and environmental dangers, 1982.
12. Douglas, M. (ed) Essays in the sociology of perception. Routledge and Kegan Paul, 1982.
13. Thompson, M. A three-dimensional model (pp 31-63) and The problem of the centre: an autonomous cosmology (pp 302-27). In Douglas, M. (ed.) Essays in the sociology of perception. Routledge and Kegan Paul, 1982.
14. Clarke, W C. Witches, floods, and wonder drugs: historical perspectives on risk management. In Schwing, R C and Albers, W A (eds) Societal risk assessment: how safe is safe enough. Plenum, 1980.

14

Risk assessment and the control of toxic substances in the workplace

CLIVE JENKINS

Introduction

We seem to be suffering at the present time from a collective amnesia about the original pressure for government intervention in the field of public health in general and occupational health in particular. Both in America and in Britain, there has been media support for the view that the cost of legislation in many fields is greater than the benefits it bestows on society as a whole. This argument at its crudest level simply regards health as an individual matter and at a more sophisticated level involves the use of such techniques as cost/benefit analysis.

Those who propagate these views are not noted for their intellectual rigour or their sense of history. However, the generalized allegation that industry is carrying some kind of unnacceptable burden remains and must be countered. Unfortunately industrialists and politicians in this country are rarely as direct as their American counterparts. The Chairman of Koppers Co., USA at a conference in 1978 said 'you and I know that the market system would not give us environmental protection, worker safety and health. They are not economic things; they add value not wealth. The only way to improve the quality of life is through intervention'. (1)

There is no evidence that business voluntarily takes into account the general health issues of society and in fact there is growing evidence to the contrary. To take a British example, we have no policy or strategy in this country for the disposal of toxic waste. This is not surprising. The Gregson Report noted 'we do not know how much hazardous waste is produced in the UK, who produces it, what it is and what happens to it' (2). Those regulations which do exist are ignored and short term financial gain takes precedence over the long term costs of dealing with land fill waste sites which will normally fall on society as a whole. The Chairman of Rechem said recently 'in the last year we have lost 15% of our chemical treatment business. Some of this is due to the recession but a lot more is due to industry switching back to land fill and cutting corners' (3).

The case for an interventionist policy has been made. The kind of strategy that is needed is a more complex matter. Britain led the world in its public health policies in the late nineteenth century, and it led in most of the important developments in occupational health. It did so on the basis that health was an issue of social, economic and political policy. I argue that these are still the central issues and that the arguments are not essentially different today from 50 years ago.

Self regulation
There is a great deal of misleading argumentation in the field of health and safety about the need for self regulation. This was a particularly fashionable phrase around the time of the Robens Report in 1972 (4). The Act which actually reached the statute book was a framework of law. 'Self Regulation' in this context does not mean that employers should be responsible for their own standards although industry spokespersons have clearly regarded this as the case. 'Greater efficiency does not mean more legislation; self regulation is equally valid in a recession'. (5)

John Locke, Director General of the Health and Safety Executive, has a rather clearer view. 'Self Regulation' in the health and safety context means that 'those who are going to be affected by health and safety Regulations and codes of Practice should be closely involved in their preparation.......Individual industries should feel a responsibility for identifying their own special problems and finding solutions..... Thirdly, in the individual workplace "self regulation" means to me that management and workers accept a responsibility for carrying out the general duties set out in the 1974 Act'. (6)

I have no quarrel with this formula except that the role of trade unions in the field of occupational health issues is a great deal more complex than the majority of safety issues. The right to know is a fundamental pre-requisite to responsible action and, in the current climate, to face a worker with a choice between work and health is again to individualize social choices which are inherently collective. A citizen of London can no more opt for a lead-free environment than a worker in Associated Octel can opt for another job in the industrial devastation of Liverpool.

The employer strategy of treating all regulations as if they were unjustified on the grounds of costs is easy to demolish. Such arguments historically would have been used to defend slavery or child labour and indeed they were. A more sophisticated approach has, therefore, been required and that has come in the form of cost/benefit analys is. In our experience of dealing with health and safety issues there are a number of very real practical problems in applying a technique which was developed essentially as a tool of economic, not social, decision-making.

The difficulty of accurately defining costs
Industry does not cost health and safety in a way which can produce agreed data. A recent NEDO report from the chemicals sector highlights the problem:

> Companies, however, are rarely able to quantify accurately the costs in this very diverse area. It is not possible, therefore to comment on the extent to which procedures and legislation act or may act as a constraint on the growth of the chemical industry.
>
> No evidence was found of economic benefits at company level comparable with financial costs; as with costs, benefits are difficult to identify and quantify, thus it should not be concluded that none exist.
>
> Accident statistics for the industry, including those produced by the Health and Safety Executive and the Chemical Industries Association, are dubious in their significance and give no indication at all of any improvement. Statistics on employee health are effectively non-existent. (7)

Trade unions have a further problem. To accept business assertions about actual costs at face value is about as credible as asking the taxman's advice on how to avoid income tax. The kind of claims that were made about the cost of controlling exposure to vinyl chloride monomer in the PVC industry adds some factual basis to suspicion (8).

I also have another reservation about costing which comes from my experience as a member of the Advisory Committee on Toxic Substances (9). At no time during my three years of membership have the employers actually been prepared to lay costs on the table and justify them. This was specifically requested in relation to the benzene standard because of the persistent generalizations about costs. No such breakdown was ever forthcoming. I draw from this the conclusion that industry is prepared to make a great deal out of exaggerated costs in generalities but rarely they are prepared to justify them.

The difficulty of quantifying benefits
How do you quantify the absence of fear from the development of a long term disease? How do you quantify an unhealthy retirement?

Nor is it the case that these risks are spread evenly over the community. To paraphrase Vic Feather who once said 'it's not that 100% of the population are 10% unemployed, it's that 10% of the population are 100% unemployed'. It is important to remember this when discusing chronic and often fatal diseases.

Our experience is that these issues do not get quantified as they are essentially unquantifiable and therefore are simply left out. They are, however, the essence of social policy and undermine the applicability of cost benefit techniques to health and safety issues.

A common scale
Any proponent of cost benefit analysis knows that costs and benefits have to be expressed on a common scale for the analysis to stand up. The problem of applying this to occupational health and safety is that those who carry the costs are rarely those who get the benefits. An enterprise is only willing to make an assessment within its own economic criteria, it does not take into account the cost, for example, to the National Health Service of chronic ill health caused by working in dusty industries.

The cost to industry and the cost to society are in different spheres and I have yet to see a system that resolves this dilemma. It is not even clear at the macro level what social costs are to be included (10).

My reservations, however, go deeper. For normal economic exchanges compensation is often as good as prevention. If you damage my car the cost to fix it is a fair exchange. Health cannot be purchased. The asbestos victims illustrate this point. It took a television programme to remind us that each asbestos related illness involves a real person (11). To criticise this on the grounds of sensationalising the issue is nonsense. The opposite is the case. Hard facts and figures immure us to the human tragedies that lie behind them. As Bill Simpson said in respect of the cancer debate 'if you cannot get emotional about your own death, I am not sure what you can get emotional about'. (12) Trade unions have accepted for some time that compensation is but a poor alternative to prevention.

While rejecting the cruder forms of the cost benefit analysis, society has to have some mechanism for deciding which policies have priority over others and how socially desirable objectives can most effectively be achieved. It brings us to the central issues of how this process should take place and the difficulties which can be involved. I think the issue of controlling chemicals in the workplace, particularly carcinogens, illustrates these difficulties.

In February, 1980, ASTMS issued a Policy Document on the Prevention of Occupational Cancer (13). The purpose of the document was primarily to inform and alert our members to what we considered a real and growing problem, but it was also to engage in the arena of public policy making.

The main principles of the policy were as follows:

(1) cancer can best be defeated through a policy of prevention, based on the fact that the disease is caused overwhelmingly by environmental cancer agents, including occupational carcinogens;

(2) cancer agents pose a hazard which is qualitatively different from that of most other toxic substances, in that:

> * there is no known safe level of exposure;
>
> * there is a long latent period between exposure and contracting the disease;
>
> * the disease is irreversible and often fatal, except in some cases such as skin cancer;
>
> * detection of susceptible individuals is not feasible.

(3) A policy of waiting to 'count the bodies' by epidemiological methods is unacceptable as the sole basis for detecting cancer agents. In addition there must be an agreed method of preventing exposure of workers to agents that can cause cancer in animals which are very active in short term tests.

(4) This detection programme needs to be backed by stringent regulation by government authorities, through:

> * a chemicals pre-testing scheme which subjects all new chemicals to cancer tests before being put on the market;
>
> > * a general cancer policy which places automatic controls on substances once they are recognised as cancer agents - to reduce exposure to such substances in the workplace to the lowest feasible level.

(5) Trades Union and employers can reach agreement locally to undertake thorough searches to check that carcinogens are not being used, or if they are found, to be substituted wherever feasible. Where substitution is impractical, then exposure must be reduced as close to zero as possible through total containment of operations (14).

I do not propose to repeat the arguments on the above points. Instead for the purposes of this seminar I propose to look at three specific areas:

> (1) Should workers representatives be involved in the assessment of risk?
>
> (2) How much cancer is caused by occupational factors?
>
> (3) What level of proof is required for the development of a prevention policy?

In order to have a reasoned debate, we must have some agreement about the use of terms and on the difference between fact and opinion. In the field of cancer policy, this has been particularly difficult and one in which we ourselves have been accused of lacking objectivity. A recent editorial in the BMJ began 'the debate in the United States concerning the likely contribution of occupational factors to the incidence of cancer and its mortality has been furious and vitriolic'. (15)

Instead of engaging in detail in this debate I would simply like to quote a recent letter to the Journal of Occupational Medicine which puts the points clearly and succinctly:

Choice of Terms Potentially Misleading
To the Editor: In a recent article, Sir Richard Doll skillfully summarized the contribution of epidemiology to the prevention of cancer (JOM 23: 601-609, 1981).

The choice of terms for the second type of application, captioned 'Determination of Socially Acceptable Hazards' is potentially misleading, and I must therefore object. In the text, Sir Richard speaks somewhat more modestly of the potential contribution: 'What epidemiology (and epidemiology alone) can do is to demonstrate the size of the risk that is associated with a particular level of exposure and therefore help to determine the level that is socially acceptable. By the illustrations of this area of application with data on possible effects of urban air pollution by benzo(a)pyrene and data on saccharin and bladder cancer he has merely chosen two controversial problems for which the existing epidemiological information shows a negligible risk. How this relates to the social acceptability of the known carcinogenic properties of the agents is far from clear. In fact, limitations of exposure are the most relevant steps toward making the risks acceptable, and the epidemiologists have had little to contribute to this process.

The determination of risk acceptability is not a scientific process, as Lowrance (1) has made clear, although all scientific work can contribute to estimation of risk. When work in toxicology finds that an agent is an animal carcinogen, but epidemiology fails to identify human risk, the issue until now has been passed on to legislators, lawyers and other policy-makers. This class of suspect agents is relatively large, and with present levels of support, epidemiology is hardly contributing to the resolution of the policy issues for reasons inherent in the field, as Sir Richard points out. Epidemiology has a distinctive and critical role to play in risk assessment, and that is what Sir Richard is describing. With respect to the prevention of occupational cancer, there are two types of problems for which epidemiology has not fulfilled its potential, and the deficiency is our own and not due to lack of support. These topics are the occurrence of other illnesses or impairment at an earlier period or with lower doses of agents known to be human carcinogens. We have been ignoring the potentiality of these sentinel reactions for the prevention of occupational cancer. Secondly, for at least 20 years we have had evidence that there were a number of occupations with excess risk of cancer, but for which the identification of agents was missing or ignored.

The implications of the first situation are that prevention of other associated diseases or impairments can have a central position in the effort to prevent cancer. The implication of the second is that both more careful evaluations are needed for the exposures of persons in occupations at high risk, and that exposures to potentially carcinogenic agents need to be reduced. Thus these somewhat neglected aspects of occupational cancer epidemiology lead to suggested improvements in epidemiological monitoring and in industrial hygienic conditions....

To me it seems ironic that Professor Doll's carefully reasoned reappraisal of the inflated estimates of the proportion of cancer associated with occupational exposures - put together to support a socially admirable goal of a more adequate Federal cancer control policy - should itself be weakened by the presumption that epidemiologists should engage in determination of what hazards are socially acceptable.

The determination of the magnitude of health risks from occupational exposures is the essential work of occupational epidemiology. The determination of how much of what kinds of risk are acceptable is a political and not a scientific task.

John R. Goldsmith, M.D.
Professor of Epidemiology
Ben Gurion University of the Negav
P.O.B. 653
Beer Sheva 84 120, Israel

(NB Professor Doll subsequently accepted the main point of Professor Goldsmith's argument.)

On this basis, therefore, I will examine the three aspects of the cancer debate that have been particularly illuminating in respect of the assessment of risk.

Should workers' representatives be involved in the assessment of risk?
In 1983 this would seem a ridiculous question embodying an outmoded paternalism irrelevant to a democratic society. The trade unions' defence of the participation of workers in the process of risk assessment is based partly on the moral rectitude of such a position and partly that workers do have practical experience that is relevant to the evaluation process. In Britain the rights of trade unions to participate in the assessment of risk are embodied in the 1974 Health and Safety at Work Act, although it must be emphasized that there are major aspects of occupational risk which do not come into this system. For example the Advisory Committee on Pesticides has no trade union representation and despite criticism by the Director General of the Health and Safety Executive (16) and vague promises from the Minister of Agriculture this remains the position at the time of writing.

Resistance to the role of trade unions is more commonly associated with single entrepreneurs than large companies which are members of modern employers' associations. What has been interesting however, in respect of the occupational cancer debate, is just how attractive the strategy of exclusion from decision making has been to employers who wish to limit controls on occupational carcinogens. Following the publication of the ASTMS Policy Document, a number of employers' associations were sufficiently concerned to orchestrate a response (17).

ASTMS has replied to these criticisms in detail and I do not propose to repeat this here but to look beyond the content of such criticisms to the strategy they embodied. The first line of defence was that cancer policy is a clinical question and must be left to the experts. This attempted to avoid the ASTMS argument that occupational cancer is not a medical problem but one which employers and unions must resolve in the workplace itself by removing and controlling carcinogens. This was backed up in the case of the Chemical Industries Association by a refusal to have anything other than a 'medical' meeting where the CIA's medical advisors would meet the trade union medical advisors. Both ASTMS and the GMBATU have consistently refused to accept this position and the CIA eventually has been forced to abandon it.

The justification for the CIA position is contained in an unpublished paper which has widely been circulated (18). It is essentially the same as the European Chemical Industry, Ecology and Toxicology Centre Monograph 'Risk Assessment of Occupational Chemical Carcinogens' (19). The basic premise of both papers is that trade unions are to be excluded as far as possible from the risk assessment and those who are exposed to hazards should have little or no say in what is an acceptable level of risk. After distinguishing 'hazard' and 'risk', the CIA suggests that each should be treated separately by special assessment groups. These groups, the CIA proposes, are to be made up of specialists 'with a high degree of expertise from a wide variety of disciplines'. Given the small number of non-industry toxicologists, it would be difficult - indeed impossible - to gather the sort of specialists who would fulfil the CIA's other criterion - that of complete impartiality.

The trade unions simply do not accept that experts employed by the chemical industry are truly 'impartial'. Such a view would fly in the face of the trade unions' experience of dealing with occupational health issues, apart from the wider debate concerning 'value free' science. Even the line these experts are expected to take is made obvious by the CIA's suggestion that the risk assessment group should be further advised on matters of economic impact and costs of alternative actions, etc. It would seem that the risk being assessed is really that of industry having to spend some money. The health workers appears to be very low on the group's intended agenda. This should come as no suprise since on page 3 of this document, the CIA state that economic considerations should 'largely determine whether the required control technology can be applied or whether the material or process will be retained in use'.

There is no mention anywhere in this document of the need to inform workers and their representatives of the hazards and risks from their work. Indeed, the CIA obviously wish to maintain maximum secrecy on this matter. They disapprove of topics being publicly discussed 'before the available data has been properly examined'. Instead the CIA proposes that the HSE should decide which chemicals should have priority for assessment. This proposal precludes not only union, but CBI involvement in this vital process. Close involvement with assessment groups composed of industrial experts would further ensure that the most important decisions were taken before the matter even reached ACTS (20). A climate of secrecy and lack of debate may suit the CIA but is hardly satisfactory for any other interested parties and is not calculated to encourage confidence.

The process of hazard and risk assessment is laid out in less parochial terms in the ECETOC paper. Instead of the two-tier process ECETOC has invented a third which would in the British context equate to the role of ACTS. These three stages are worth quoting in full:

> *Hazard Identification.* The aim of this first stage in risk assessment is to establish qualitatively whether a carcinogenic hazard exists. A chemical is classified, according to the evidence concerning its carcinogenic potential, as a Proven, Putative or Questionable Human Carcinogen.
>
> To achieve this classification, information on carcinogenic potential needs to be developed in a sequence of steps as described in section B.2.
>
> Such classification is essential for identifying Proven and Putative carcinogens for which risk assessment is necessary. Classification as Questionable in the early stages of Hazard Identification indicates that more work is required to permit a re-classification into one of the other classes, or a decision that for practical purposes the chemical should be considered as a non-carcinogen for humans - see section B.1.
>
> *Risk Estimation.* Once a carcinogenic hazard (i.e. situation with a potential for causing cancer) has been identified it is necessary to quantify as far as possible the carcinogenic potency of the substance and the factors relevant to human exposure at the workplace. By relating these, the risk is characterised in as quantitative a way as possible. Both the collection of the necessary information and the characterisation of the risk are considered to constitute the Risk Estimation stage.
>
> Risk Estimation is feasible only for Proven and Putative Human Chemical Carcinogens because by definition there is insufficient evidence for chemicals in the Questionable class. In making a Risk Estimation there is a practical

requirement to distinguish between carcinogens of widely-differing potency in spite of the many limitations in the expression of such potency. This can be achieved by a group of experienced scientists capable of assessing the various factors involved. By relating the potency of a carcinogen to that of other Human or Putative carcinogens it can be categorised as of high, medium or low potency. This process is described in section C.1. Factors necessary for assessing human exposure to the chemical at the workplace, also necessary in Risk Estimation, are detailed in section C.2. It is emphasised that very rarely is sufficient evidence available to enable a Risk Estimation to be expressed numerically in such terms as '1 in 10^6 risk of cancer at an exposure of 10 ppm'. The question therefore becomes more one of expert judgement than of mathematics. This is why the term Risk Estimation is used.

Hazard Identification and Risk Estimation are tasks for an experienced group of toxicologists and other experts from all necessary disciplines.

Risk Limitation : the information from the Risk Estimation stage is considered, together with important additional factors such as the social and economic consequences, technological feasibility, etc. and final recommendation for an exposure level and/or working conditions is made.

This is a task for a group comprising representatives of the parties ultimately concerned in implementing the recommendations made to control the risk, plus experts from the Risk Estimation group.

This is a highly complicated formulation but one which if looked at carefully removes a substantial part of risk assessment into the scientific arena, and therefore under the control, in this context, of the company experts. Expert judgement comes to the fore and social and economic judgement retreats to the final stage where even then the experts will be involved. The CIA and ECETOC positions could be seen as irrelevant if they were not part of a more general climate of opinion to exclude trade unions from the decision-making process. I hope I will be forgiven for saying that it is tiresome for each generation of trade union leaders to fight the same battles about basic representational rights.

How much cancer is occupational?
There are in my experience two very effective ways of resisting legislative action. Firstly, to ensure that no data is effectively collected so that the debate can go on forever as to whether or not a problem really exists. This is readily illustrated by my previous quotation on toxic waste. It has been equally true in relation to the cancer debate. At the present time there is no requirement on companies to keep records for epidemiological purposes; there is no requirement to reveal information if such studies are in fact done.

I hope this situation will be remedied in the near future by the introduction of detailed regulations for the Control of Substances Hazardous to Health (21). However, what I wish to point out here is that industry lobbies have delayed and delayed effective regulation by straightforward opposition to collecting data that could be publicly available (22).

The second strategy is to collect the data in a way that downgrades the problem or in more extreme cases makes it disappear! An example of this is to use the Industrial Injuries Prescribed Diseases lists as an indication of the amount of occupational cancer. Thus you set up a system which defines which cases of occupational cancer are compensatable and you then use that as a figure for the estimate of *actual* occupationally related cancers. Would that all problems were solved so easily!

It is important to note that not all problems of paucity of data can be laid at the door of employers. While our cancer registries are the envy of the world, they have severe limitations for the purposes of identifying occupational cancer.

The lack of appreciation of the importance of records and their linkage in the identification of the toxic effects of man-made chemicals means that the processing of medical records, the maintainance of disease registers and the training of skilled medical records personnel all have low priority in the competition for resources. In times of economic stringency, as at present, the actual continued existence of the National Cancer Registers in England and Wales and the morbidity data collecting system in Scotland are threatened.

Equally important as a discouragement to further developments in this field is the ambiguity of the Government's approach to medical record linkage. A clear statement of the propriety and importance of this work is urgently needed together with a code of practice to define the proper limits of the use of these techniques in the interests of health with proper safeguards to privacy and legal protection for the custodians of the data (23).

Nothing illustrates the difficulties of interpretation of data in the cancer debate as the estimates of cancer due to certain causes. The Califano Report had just been produced when the ASTMS Report was in its final stages (24). This report has been criticised by independent academics as well as industry spokespersons and seems to have caused one of the bitterest scientific controversies in recent years.

Estimates of cancer due to occupational causes vary considerably. Wynder and Gom in 1977 gave estimates of between 1-10% but detailed documentation of methodology was not available (25). Higginson and Muir 1979 used a modified 'site specific attributable risk technique' but again gave little detailed documentation (26). Cole in 1977 estimated 15% in men and 5% in women (27). This was essentially an industry by industry response but again based very much on estimates. Fox and Adelstein 1979 said 12% using a technique called social class standardization (28).

All of these estimates were criticized by the Birdbord et al Report on the following grounds:

1. Incomplete data.

2. The fallacy of 'one effect - one cause' explanations (eg attributing lung cancer to smoking even when clear occupational exposure agents such as asbestos was a contributory factor).

3. Latent period, age and duration of exposure (previous epidemiological studies have often uncovered only a fraction of total deaths attributable to a cancer agent).

4. Changes in exposure patterns.

The Report also points out that previous approaches tried to estimate the proportion of present cases of cancer attributable to exposure in the past - but a far more relevant question is the contribution of present exposure to future cancer incidence (29).

The Birdbord paper tried to get round these problems in a number of ways which have been criticised in some detail. 'The method used for projection of the future annual risks among current employees in each of six industries was to multiply the number of millions of workers currently employed there, *irrespective of their actual duration or degree of exposure* (which will be negligible in many cases) by the % excess risks of cancer that have been observed by special epidemiological study in the United States or elsewhere among a few hundred or a few thousand workers who have been heavily exposed for many years to the agent of interest'. (30) Doll and Peto then went on to produce their estimate of 2% - 8%. Their approach has been criticised on the grounds that it depends too much on epidemiology (epidemiology having identified less than 60 substances as carcinogenic to humans) (31). In addition they have been criticised for their interpretation of cancer trends. These criticisms are summarized in the quotation below:

> My colleagues and I have reached three pertinent conclusions on cancer mortality for sites associated with occupation for males in the past decade. First, while the proportion of older men dying from *all causes* has declined, the proportion dying from certain cancers has increased. Multiple myeloma and cancers of the lung and based sharply in those aged 55 to 84 - at least 50 percent for those between 75 and 84. Second, other cancers known to be associated with occupation (kidney, oesophagus, and liver) have also increased in older men. Finally, some cancers associated with cigarette smoking have declined (bladder, pancreas, buccal cavity and pharynx), while others have increased (lung, oesophagus and kidney).
>
> These findings do not present a simple picture. Some of the declines in mortality reflect improved treatment, especially for bladder cancer, which is now among the curable cancers. Some of the increases may be artefacts, resulting from increased use of high technology for diagnoses. In addition, the cancers associated with cigarette smoking also are associated with occupation and (in some cases) alcohol and nutrition. Undeniably, as Doll and Peto indicate, cigarette smoking remains the chief preventable cause of most cancers. It is also responsible for a host of other public health problems, ranging from heart disease to fires to low birth weight. But our data suggest that the real contribution of occupational and environmental exposures remains an important research question that cannot be readily resolved by examining national cancer rates. (32)

If you read these articles on cancer estimates, all the authors in fact acknowledge that the estimates are unreliable. 'Information which would *allow* a barest quantitative assessment of risks....... is for the most part lacking'. (33)

No doubt the protagonists will continue to debate the issue and perhaps the most diplomatic contribution to the debate came surprisingly from the Office of Carcinogen Identification and Classification of OSHA; a somewhat beleaguered outpost in the current US regulatory climate.

> All of these reports have served a very useful purpose in stimulating interest towards identifying areas of emphasis for allocation of resources for future research into the aetiology of environmental cancer. However, there is no sound basis upon which to determine on a quantitative level, the contribution of such broad categories to the total cancer burden. In our opinion, further quantitative estimates using data currently available will serve only to divert much needed resources that could be used in more meaningful activities. If society chooses to seriously embark on an effort to quantify environmental causes of cancer, there is a need to commence activity for establishing criteria and data that would be necessary to answer the question in the future. (34)

I interpret this and similar statements as a truce among the academics. They are essentially saying that the kind of information which the policy makers require is unavailable. Is the answer then simply to delay action until such proof is available? This leads on to what I consider to be the most important aspect of the whole debate. What level of proof is required for the development of preventative policy?

The development of health and safety legislation in Britain has been heavily weighted in favour of initiatives on safety rather than health. Some of the reasons for this are clear enough. Safety is more visible, more immediate but the development and the nature of legislation itself has also been a factor. Under the Factories Acts, there is a clear and unequivocal duty on employers to guard machinery. In legal cases it has been held that if an injury occurred, then almost by definition, the machine has not been properly guarded.

Section 63 of the same Act lays down a duty to be kept as far as practicable in relation to the removal of dust and fumes from the workplace. The duty to guard has been an endless basis for effective prosecution by the Inspectorate and our high standard of machinery guarding derives from it. On the other hand, there have been a few successful prosecutions under Section 63. This has been almost entirely due to the level of proof required. A successful prosecution under Section 63 requires the prosecution to prove *beyond all reasonable doubt* that the substance involved is injurious to health. I doubt if, by this criteria, smoking would stand convicted. The estimate of future *potential* risk does not fit easily into this level of legal proof.

Exactly the same problem faces those who are trying to develop a preventative strategy in the field of toxic substances at work. This problem is particularly acute where reliable human data is absent. This is almost universally the case with respect to carcinogens. The debate on acceptable proof has become whether or not we can act on animal data or whether we have to have evidence of *actual* human disease. A policy of waiting to collect human evidence has a certain Alice in Wonderland quality. As the Queen said to Alice: 'Sentence now verdict later'.

There are a number of reasons why the epidemiological method is inappropriate in a strategy for the prevention of occupational cancer.

Epidemiology cannot identify relatively low levels of risk. Few epidemiological studies have been adequate to detect anything smaller than a 50% increase in the cancer incidence compared with the general population. The main arguments are:

1. The period between exposure and the onset of the disease can be anything up to 50 years. As strategy for prevention this has obvious drawbacks.

2. Very rarely are workers exposed to single substances and the pursuit of a single carcinogen is often a hopeless task. A needle in a haystack is a useful metaphor for a carcinogen in a dyestuff plant or a carcinogen in the rubber industry.

3. In order to establish exposure levels a large amount of data has to be available. There have, of course, to be personal records. Many or all of the basic information sources are missing.

For these reasons, the defence of epidemiological studies as the determining tool of a cancer prevention policy fits well into the strategy described previously. If you make sure the evidence is never going to be available you can delay regulations for ever.

It should not, of course, be assumed that we take the view that all animal data are relevant. (One of the most positive developments in the cancer field has been the development of criteria for animal studies.) Nor that all epidemiology where it does exist should be dealt with uncritically. The Trade unions have been too often on the receiving end of the use of non—positive as opposed to negative epidemiology to overlook this aspect. Today, we are more frequently told some or other study shows no excess of risk and I suppose this is a slight improvement on when we were told there was no study because there was no risk.

I would also like to welcome recent developments in the International Agency for Cancer Research (35). Their tentative steps into the field of quantitative risk assessment may well be a useful contribution to the debate. However, to date, the scientific principles of the OSHA policy remain the basis for any preventative policy. These can be summarised as follows:

* Properly designed and conducted tests using appropriate animal species (eg rats and mice) are accepted as valid ways to identify chemical substances that may cause cancer in humans. In nearly all cases, chemicals that cause cancer in humans have been found to cause cancer in small rodents.

* Established test protocols, which include administration of high doses, sometimes by a route different from the expected human exposure route, are appropriate and scientifically valid methods for identifying potential carcinogens in humans. The intrinsic carcinogenic character of a chemical substance is independent of dose level. High doses simply make this characteristic easier to discern in a test stuation. Chemical carcinogens tested by one route usually produce cancers when tested by other routes as well.

* Induction of benign tumours is accepted as an indication of carcinogenic potential of a substance unless definitive evidence shows the substance incapable of inducing malignant tumours. Some tumours pass through benign stages as they progress to malignancy, and some chemicals may produce benign and malignant tumours.

* Methods do not now exist for determining a safe threshold level of exposure to carcinogens. Uncertainties in the dose-response relationship between specific exposures and cancer risk, unknown factors that influence individual susceptability to cancer, and unpredictable interactions among cancer-causing agents prevent determination of safe levels for human exposure to a carcinogen. Any exposure, however small, is regarded as an addition to the total carcinogenic risk.

* Methods now available for quantifying the estimated human risks from a given exposure to a potential carcingen can provide only approximations of the actual risk (36).

'Sentence now verdict later'
It should therefore be fairly clear that a level of proof beyond all reasonable doubt is only another way of avoiding regulation on a problem. Nor has the 'medicalization' of ill health been particularly useful in advancing public health policies. This debate is, of course, much wider than occupational health. From Illich to Ian Kennedy, the role of doctors in the *prevention* of disease is under attack.

When I have been reading the flood of recent papers on the subject, I recall the statement made by Dr Richard Bates at the OSHA hearings on their cancer policy.

A classical episode in the history of disease prevention took place in London in 1854. An epidemic of cholera occurred in the neighbourhood around Broad Street. John Snow, the hero of the story, studied the habits of the victims and found that almost all obtained their water from the well on Broad Street. Swift action was taken: the pump was closed down and the epidemic rapidly subsided. This disease was caused by exposure to the bacterium *Vibrio cholerae*. One can imagine the reaction that might occur today if it were proposed to close down the pump on the basis of evidence of the kind obtained by John Snow. Many scientists would point out that it had not been conclusively demonstrated that the water was the cause of the disease. They would be troubled because of the lack of satisfactory theoretical knowledge to explain how the water could have caused the disease. Further more, other habits of those who had become ill had not been adequately investigated, so it would not be possible to rule out other causes of the disease. The scientists would have been correct. Others would have pointed out that some members of the community who drank from the Broad Street well had not succumbed to cholera. Thus, even if there were something wrong with the water, there must be other factors involved, and if we could control these we would not have to be concerned about the water. These conclusions are also correct. Some who consumed water from the Broad Street well would have objected to closing it because the taste of water from other wells was not as agreeable. Finally, if the pump had been owned by an individual who sold the water, he would certainly have protested against closing down his business on the basis of inconclusive evidence of hazard.

This story illustrates a number of points that need to be kept in mind as we examine the proposed carcinogen policy of the Occupational Safety and Health Administration. First, if human disease and deaths are to be prevented, it is often necessary to control exposure for which there is some evidence of hazard before that evidence has reached the point that scientists would universally regard as conclusive. The alternative, to continue exposure until there is conclusive evidence of human hazard, is a form of human experimentation that our society finds increasingly unacceptable.

Second, development of a disease in any individual is the result of complex interactions of a variety of factors including his or her genetic susceptibility; environmental influences on the person's state of susceptibility that may include such things as exposure to other harmful agents in the environment, the person's state of nutrition, age and general health; and finally the level and extent of exposure to specific disease causing agents. These principles hold true for cholera; not all who drank from the Broad Street well developed cholera. These principles also apply to cancer induction; cancer develops in susceptible individuals exposed to carcinogenic agents.

Third, the incidence of disease in a population can be reduced either by reducing exposure to specific causative agents or through general or specific measures that reduce the level of susceptibility of the population to the causative agents. The state of our knowledge about the specific disease determines which measures can be applied most successfully at any particular time in history. During John Snow's time, removing the supply of contaminated water was the most feasible approach. Today, cholera can also be controlled through immunization and mortality can be reduced through specific therapy. During John Snow's time, however, the latter options were not available. Control of tuberculosis has resulted as much from better nutrition and improved living conditions as it resulted from hospitalization of diseased individuals. These general health measures increased resistance of the population to the disease agent. More specific immunization techniques against tuberculosis have been developed, but their effectiveness has been a matter of considerable debate for many years.

With cancer, the major method of prevention available to us today is to prevent exposure to chemicals and radiations capable of inducing the disease. (37)

Towards a social strategy of risk assessment
One of the most insidious aspects of the cost/benefit fashion in the assessment of risk is the attempt to equate one type of risk with another across a whole range of different hazards. Tables are produced comparing the risk of crashing in an aircraft with crossing the road and with working in a chemical factory. One of the minor problems with this kind of assessment is that it concentrates on mortality rather than morbidity.

Quality of life still remains more important than quality of death. However, the fallacy is much more profound. It was aptly illustrated by the red lollipop controversy and the American Cancer Society. The dye in the red lollipops was a suspect carcinogen and the Society which was selling them for promotional purposes was asked to stop. The Society replied that as they were still on the market, ie government had not banned the dye, this was perfectly alright. Not so, declared the protagonists, the Society would not dream of raising money by selling cigarettes. I am indebted for this little anecdote to Barry Commoner who goes on as follows to make the following substantive point:

> Suppose we compare the costs of a regulatory action that might be taken against cigarettes or red lollipops - banning them. Banning cigarettes would wipe out a $6 billion industry (in annual sales), whereas banning even all uses of Red Dye No. 40 would eliminate sales of only a few million dollars per year. Clearly, the social costs of banning red lollipops are much smaller than the costs of banning cigarettes. But this fact would, of course, be a palpably illogical basis for action, since cigarettes are more dangerous. The logical fault is obvious: In a risk/benefit assessment what should be compared is risk and benefit associated with the same substance, not risk (or benefit) of Substance A with the risk (or benefit) of Substance B (38).

The whole history of control of toxic substances and indeed drugs and pesticides has been to avoid the issue of social use of particular products. Yet I cannot see ultimately how any reasonable strategy can avoid the issue indefinitely. Nor is this an issue which leaves union interests unscathed. We may ban lead in petrol, but who in the name of wider social good will confront easily the workers made redundant as a consequence? In order to make any policy socially acceptable there has to be some allocation of costs.

I must argue finally that economic criteria have little initial place in a policy of controlling toxic substances at work. We seem to have forgotten that the idea of right and wrong is also a relevant criterion of social judgement. There is a straightforward proposition which states that workers should not become ill as a result of their work. Furthermore, hazards in the workplace are often different from other hazards in that they are essentialy preventable. Nobody knows where a preventative strategy for breast cancer would start; on the other hand we do know an effective strategy for the prevention of mesothelioma, that is by banning the use of asbestos.

Risks taken at work are not voluntary and it is a great mistake to base any social policy on the assumption that they are. Nor do I actually think that a great many 'voluntary' matters such as bad diets and smoking are quite as voluntary as is ocasionally pretended. I would, therefore, like to conclude with a plea that we abandon trying to rest upon inadequate science as a basis for social policy; that we act on the evidence that is available in the context of clear moral values; that society does have a duty to protect us from the untrammelled effects of the free market approach. Long may the John Snows of this world continue to act.

Could the unions be wearing his mantle?

References

1. Quoted in 'Costs and benefits vs the right thing to do'. Allied Industrial Worker p 10, (July 1982).
2. Expert witness to the House of Lords Select Committee on Science and Technology. Quoted in Ambio 2, 53, 1982.
3. Coleman, Chairman of Rechem, quoted in New Scientist, p 628, 11 March, 1982.
4. Robens Report. Report of the Committee on Safety and Health at Work, Cmnd 5034, 1970-1972.
5. Eberlie, D. Health Safety and Social Affairs Directorate, Confederation of British Industry, quoted in Protection, p 12, June 1982.
6. Locke, J. Interviewed in the Safety Practitioner, p 5-6, February 1983.
7. Chemicals EDC. Industrial Review Health and Safety and Environment. A document for discussion, NEDO, 1981.
8. ASTMS. The prevention of occupational cancer. An ASTMS policy document, p 13, 1980.
9. ACTS is the Committee of the Health and Safety Commission which formulates standards for the control of toxic substances in the workplace.
10. Unpublished critique by ASTMS of HSC discussion document: cost/benefit assessment of health safety and pollution controls. HMSO.
11. Alice, a fight for life. A Yorkshire TV documentary shown on 20 July, 1982.
12. Personal exchange.
13. ASTMS. The prevention of occupational cancer. An ASTMS policy document. 1980.
14. Health and Safety Information. ASTMS Series No 11. Prevention of occupational cancer again. 1981.
15. British Medical Journal, *283*, 1421, 1981.
16. Nature, *286*, 1980.
17. Health and Safety Information. ASTMS Series No 11. Prevention of occupational cancer again. 1981.
18. CIA. The control of occupational carcinogens. CIA position paper, 1981.
19. ECETOC. Monograph No 3. Risk assessment of occupational chemical carcinogens. Brussels, 1982.
20. ACTS is the Committee of the Health and Safety Commission which formulates standards for the control of toxic substances in the workplace.
21. As a result of the EEC Framework Directive for the control of substances hazardous to health, the HSC has had to accept that the 1974 Health and Safety at Work Act is inadequate legisation for the control of occupational ill health. This was recognised by Robens some 12 years ago and has been a repeated trade union assertion in the intervening period.
22. The experience of ASTMS in trying to get access to records, both medical and personal is considerable, and not particularly successful. Our experience of the Employment Medical Advisory Service has been little better than our experience with several major companies. Irrelevant issues of confidentiality are raised which might be perfectly proper in a clinical situation but irrelevant to epidemiology where personal details are excluded.
23. Acheson, E D. Record linkage and the identification of long term environmental hazards. Long Term Hazards from Environmental Chemicals. The Royal Society, 177, 1979.
24. The Califano report is referred to in other papers as the OSHA report or Birdbord et al (1978). It was never actually published but submitted at OSHA's public hearings on occupational cancer policy.
25. Wynder, E L and Gom, G B. Contribution of the environment to cancer incidence: an epidemiological exercise. JNCI, *58*, 825-832, 1977.
26. Higginson, J and Muir, C S. Environmental carcinogens. JNCI, *60*, 1291-1298, 1979.
27. Cole, P. Cancer, and occupation. Cancer 3, 1788-1791, 1977.
28. Fox, A J and Adelstein, Am, J Epidem Community Health, *32*, 73-78, 1978.
29. Stallones, R A and Downs, T. A critical review of estimates of the fraction of cancer in the US related to occupational factors. University of Texas School of Public Health, Houston, 1978.
30. Doll, R and Peto, R. The causes of cancer. Oxford Medical Publications, 1981.
31. Davis, D L. Estimating cancer causes: problems in methodology, production and trends. Banbury Report of Quantification of Occupational Cancer, Cold Spring Harbor Laboratory, 1981.
32. Davis, D L. Workplace cancer: the case against complacency. Environmental Law Institute, Washington, DC, 1982.
33. Doll, R and Peto, R. The causes of cancer. Oxford Medical Publications, 1981.
34. Infante, P F et al. The contribution of occupation to environmental cancers. Paper presented at the annual meeting of the American Public Health Association, November 1982.
35. IARC. *29*, 1982.
36. Toxic chemicals and public protection. A report to the President by the Toxic Substances Strategy Committee, 1980.
37. Federal Register, *45*, 5008-5009, No 15, 22.1.80.
38. Commoner, B. Comparing apples to oranges: risk of cost/ benefit analysis. Science for the People. Cambridge, Mass. 1980.

PART 4

Societal Implications & Governmental Attitudes

15
Regulation of low-level carcinogenic risk in foods: the United States view

ROBERT J SCHEUPLEIN

In his letter accompanying the completed National Academy of Sciences report on *Food Safety Policy: Scientific and Societal Considerations,* Dr Philip Handler, then President of the National Academy was led to describe the risk from dietary use of saccharin as the 'risk of a risk'.

I'm not sure what damage such a description does to some of the finely honed definitions of risk that are preferred by experts, but I find the phrase quite congenial because it aptly conveys the sense of uncertainty that underlies determinations of food-borne risk and that may undermine regulatory decisions no matter how carefully crafted they may be. This morning I would like to discuss some of the issues surrounding the regulation of low-level cancer risks from foods, food additives and contaminants in foods. The views are my own and do not represent an official FDA view, although they do reflect much of the current thinking of individuals within the agency. I hope that all of you realize that I cannot give you the current, official, US view on risk assessment. There is no official view! There are 5 major regulatory agencies concerned with the various sources of chemical risk in the US:

FDA - (Food, Drugs, Cosmetics and Medical Devices)
USDA - (Agricultural Products)
EPA - (The Environment)
OSHA - (The Workplace)
CPSC - (Consumer Products)

There are also the NCI and the NIP (National Toxicology Programme) which deal directly with cancer cure and prevention, the National Academy of Sciences, which is often called on to advise both the agencies and the Congress. There is the Executive Office of the President, which through OSIP (Office of Science and Technology Policy) presents the administration view, and finally and really, the most important, the Congress and the courts. A current, official government viewpoint would, if it existed, be some sort of a procedural amalgam of all of these.

There is no US overlord of risk assessment. But it would not be true to imply that there are no common threads in all of these viewpoints and that no efforts have been made to construct a uniform consensus based on a common set of principles. Such efforts have been made - the latest is by the National Academy of Sciences, just published.

It makes a couple of major points:

1. *First* it says that risk assessment and risk evaluation or the consideration of risk management alternatives, should be carefully and firmly distinguished.

2. *Second* it recognizes that risk assessment itself is laden with 'so-called scientific' judgements that are in effect inferential in nature.

3. *Third* it calls for the development of uniform inference guidelines for all federal regulatory agencies.

4. And *finally* it calls for no radical changes in the current organizational arrangements for performing risk-assessments; they will continue to be conducted within the separate agencies, ie the NAS recognizes the benefits of having agency experts familiar with the specific regulatory problems of their agencies available to the risk-assessment process.

These recommendations have grown out of public and congressional dissatisfaction with various agencies recent policies on dealing with carcinogens. I hope I can help put some of these issues in perspective by taking a look at the history of the regulation of carcinogens in food, which was the earliest area of official concern, and until recently, the most controversial.

Historical review of carcinogen regulation
Prior to the enactment of the Delaney Clause as part of the Food Additive Amendments of 1958, carcinogens were regulated under those provisions of the FD & C act having to do with 'Poisonous and deleterious substances' in food under different standards depending on the circuumstances of their entry into the food supply.

The 'ordinarily injurious' standard (Sec. 402(A) (1)) applied to natural constituents of foods, for example to solanine in potatoes, vitamin A in liver of polar bears or large fish and to capsaicin in red pepper. The 'may render injurious' standard (Sec. 402(A) (1)), a stiffer standard, was applied to added constituents. And finally, added substances, that were either 'necessary in the production of food' or were 'unavoidable by good manufacturing practices' were eligible for tolerance setting (Sec. 406). Aflatoxin and PCBs are, respectively, good examples. These standards were applicable to all food ingredients including those that presented a risk of cancer as well as any logical risk.

In the 1950s, two artificial sweeteners (Dulcin and P-4000) and also coumarin were prohibited under these provisions. I want to make a special point about these statutory provisions. You will notice that the categories they define are traditional foods, food additives and contaminants and are not distinguished on the basis of the risk anticipated from the use of these substances. Rather the FD&C Act acknowledges the public perception of the needs met and the benefits provided by various foods and food constituents. FDA believes, by and large, that Congress has incorporated this perception faithfully into the statute.

Under the Act, FDA is empowered, in effect, to permit a possibly higher level of risk for natural food substances that the public has used for generations than for new or synthetic substances added to improve food processing or to provide greater convenience, aesthetic appeal or shelf life. While these statutory provisions invite inconsistent treatment of comparable risk, FDA would be reluctant to suggest abandoning the statutory recognition of the traditional public and Congressional perception of need and benefit in favour of a regulatory scheme, based primarily on risk, which could result in the banning of ordinary foods.

The original triad of provisions has been amended several times since 1938 - each time to separate out for active regulatory attention a broad class of added substances. The Pesticide Residues Amendment of 1954 required the registration of pesticides. The Food Additives Amendment of 1958 established a licensure scheme, similar in concept to that for pesticide residues, for substances added to formulated foods or for substances used in packaging that become or can 'reasonably be expected'to become components of food. I should point out however, that carcinogens are covered quite differently in the two categories. Low level uses of pesticides are permitted if they do not cause 'any unreasonable risk to man or the environment'. Two important exceptions were made that reflect the 'perception of benefits' argument mentioned previously. Substances 'generally recognized as safe' by qualified experts - an exception embracing a large number of substances such as sugar, and salt were exempted and other substances sanctioned for use in food by USDA or FDA prior to 1958, were in effect 'grandfathered'.

In 1960 colour additive amendments required that substances used to colour foods, drugs, and cosmetics be precleared like food additives. Finally, the animal drug amendments of 1962 added new animal drugs to the growing list of additives requiring affirmative FDA approval prior to marketing. So by the 1960s the Act embodied a generalized 3-tiered safety standard that permitted greater 'risk' for substances of greater perceived value or for substances that were necessary in the appropriate processing of food or unavoidably present.

These categories have served quite well until recent times. In addition to providing a means by which the accepted benefits of food substances are considered and subjected accordingly to different safety standards, they also simplify the regulatory process. Since the initial value judgement on the relative benefit of food substances, ie the initial categorization, was made by Congress through the political process, the appropriate regulatory tracks are fixed as a matter of law. Thus much of the controversy that can occur with risk-benefit decision making, particularly when one attempts to weigh economic and social benefits against health risks, has been avoided. This brings up a point worth making. If regulatory decisions at least in the US are to be broadly acceptable, agencies must not be called upon to make fundamental risk-benefit value judgements outside of their statutory mandate. When an agency is free to enforce its own subjective value judgement in determining what is an 'acceptable risk' it has broken free from the legitimate influences it requires and that should emanate from established law and policy.

Carcinogens in the food supply got special attention for the first time in 1958 as a part of the Food Additives Amendment. Subsequently similar provisions were added to the Colour Additive Amendments of 1960 (Sec. 706(B) the Animal Drug Amendments of 1968 (Sec. 512(D) (1) (H)). The basic thrust of each clause is similar - to prevent the addition to food of any substance shown to induce cancer in man or laboratory animals. At the time of its enactment the FDA, although it did not want the clause for several reasons, did not believe it would be too troubling. FDA felt mainly that the clause was redundant and that it was not about to admit carcinogens into the food supply in any case. And for about twenty years this was an accurate prediction. The question of dose was not ignored, it was discussed at the hearings and explicitly considered in the testimony of the Secretary of Health, Education and Welfare who endorsed the conclusion of a National Cancer Institute Report:

> No one at this time can tell how much or how little of a carcinogen would be required to produce cancer in any human being, or how long it would take the cancer to develop.

Colour additives : Hearings on H.R. 7624 and S2197. Before the House, Comm. on Interstate and Foreign Commerce, 86th Cong. 2nd Sess. 61 (1969).

He went on to state:

> We have no basis for asking Congress to give us discretion to establish a safe tolerance for a substance which definitely has been shown to produce cancer when added to the diet of animals. We simply have no basis in which such discretion could be exercised because no one can tell us with any assurance at all how to establish a safe dose of any cancer *producing substance*.

The statement was made against the background of knowledge that existed at the time. I have retrieved a condensed version of what that knowledge was considered to imply in those days:

> 1. Although 'cancer can be caused by extraneous agents, not all members of the exposed population will develop cancer. Those who are most susceptible can be identified only by experience.'

> 2. 'Even a powerful carcinogen requires weeks or months to elicit cancer in mice or rats and probably requires years in man.'

> 3. 'No change need be recognizable in the organ or tissue destined to become cancerous before the cancer itself.'

> 4. 'Experience in the laboratory does not predict unequivocally the reaction of humans to the same agent. On the other hand, those few chemicals and physical agents known to produce cancer in man, with the possible exception of inorganic arsenical compounds, have elicited cancers in animals.'

> 5. 'No one at this time can tell how much or how little of a carcinogen would be required to produce cancer in any human being, or how long it would take the cancer to develop.'

> 6. 'The effect of certain chemical carcinogens can be markedly increased by other compounds with little or no carcinogenic power.'

> 7. 'The accumulated evidence suggests the irreversibility of the cancerous response once it has been initiated and further suggests a cumulative effect.'

> 8. 'The most potent carcinogens, by their very strength, are almost sure to be discovered clinically. It is assuredly the less potent carcinogens that seem most important in human cancer and provide the real problem for evaluation. A major objective of experimental carcinogenesis is, therefore, the *bioassay* for the presence of weak carcinogens.'

> 9.'Chemical configuration alone cannot be used to predict the ability of a new compound to produce cancer.'

> 10. 'Possession (by a substance) of a biological effect, known to be associated with a particular type of cancer production, may be of importance in assessing potential carcinogenicity. Examples are: Oestrogenicactivity, goitrogenic activity, production of liver cirrhosis.'

These comprised the central principles concerning the prediction of carcinogenic response, as understood at the time. I think that most oncologists would agree it is still a fair statement of what we believe to be true today. There would be some modifications and additions. However, at least some experts believe No. 5 in particular is overstated, incomplete and perhaps inadvertantly misleading. Most experts believe cancer risk from exposure to a carcinogen decreases with decreasing dose.

Progress has been made regarding the importance of basic alterations in DNA to the cancer process. The existence of DNA repair mechanisms has been established in some systems at low doses. The basic question is: Have the past 21 years produced sufficient understanding of the carcinogenic process and in the means of evaluating carcinogenic risk so that discretion can be exercised in establishing tolerances? I believe it is time for a re-examination of these issues in the light of present knowledge. I think there are at least three lines of inquiry to examine.

1. Can we now establish tolerances for carcinogens with some confidence?

2. Should we not take into account in any absolute proscription against carcinogens the unavoidable levels of these and other carcinogens in the environment?

3. Have we really recognized the impact of the inherently increasingly severe proscription against carcinogenic substances that is built into such statutory provisions as the Delaney Clause?

In 1977, FDA in a proposal designed to fill in the interstices of the statute regulating animal drug residues, outlined a procedure for establishing tolerances for carcinogens (F.R., Vol. 42, No. 35, Tuesday, Feb. 22, 77, Criteria Procedures for Evaluating Assays for Carcinogenic Residues). Animal drug residues were selected for this because Congress in the Animal Drug Amendments of 1962 virtually repealed the Delaney Clause, at least in the absolutist sense, for these additives and left the agency the dilemma of how to consistently implement the provision.

The DES proviso was an exemption from the Delaney Clause because it directed the regulation of animal drug residues through a requirement that 'no residue'of the drug be found in the animal by a method of examination considered appropriate by the Secretary. It thus, in effect, permitted residues below the sensitivity of that method. The FDA expanded this concept by arguing that 'no residue' was best interpreted to mean 'no significant risk' from the residue, as this allowed taking into account the differing potencies of carcinogens. The current version of the SOM, as the document came to be called, uses an insignificant risk level of 1 in a million over a lifetime and generally requires the very conservative 'linear extrapolation'.

It should be emphasized that risk-assessment is permissible in this instance because the statute for animal additives contains the DES proviso - there is no similar exemption for direct food or colour additives.

The next issue to reconsider is that of cancer 'background'. When the Congress last considered cancer policy relative to food constituents some 20 years ago - the extent of the low- level carcinogenic contamination of our natural food supply was not appreciated. Polycyclic hydrocarbons, carcinogenic mycotoxins, nitrosamines, goitrogens, naturally occurring oestrogens are widely dispersed in our natural food supply. Many others are present in low concentrations in traditional food, spices and flavours.

When the risk from these unregulated substances is estimated by current extrapolation techniques it far exceeds current 'insignficant' cancer risk levels for regulated substances. Recently FDA, in its regulation of a hair dye containing the animal carcinogen lead acetate, was persuaded of the insignificance of the cancer risk to consumers in no small part because of the fact that the amount of lead absorbed was insignificant in comparison to the much higher background levels present in our bodies from varied and uncontrollable exposures.

Finally on the issue of the increasing severity of a 'no risk'philosophy embodied in our statutes. When the Delaney Clause was enacted, routine analytical sensitivity was somewhat less than 1 ppm. Gas chromatology was in its infancy; gas-liquid chromatography, specific ion electrodes, atomic absorption and other more exquisite analytical techniques were either not yet invented or not then widely applied. These new techniques have pushed the frontiers of chemical detection to the part per trillion level and have extended the range of food substances, solvent, food contact or packaging material, etc.... that may eventually come under the prohibition of the Delaney Clause.

Time, in fact, seems to be running out rapidly, for if section 409 were to be fully enforced it is difficult to imagine how many of the food packaging materials in current use could remain regulated or regulatory agencies would deal with contaminants in food, food additives and colour additives, etc., or how we can undress the probable outcome of devastating toxicologic findings on natural and synthetic flavours and spices.

It is not at all clear that 86th Congress recognized that substances that were then considered safe under the ambit of the Delaney Clause would in future years irresistibly come under its ban simply as a consequence of better detection methods.

16
The acceptable risk
and the Council of Europe

GILLY GOBINET

Introduction

One of the roles of the Council of Europe (1), a 21-member inter-governmental organisation, is to promote public health and encourage the harmonisation of national health legislations. But what happens when national views on the same particular issue differ to the extent that an associated risk is considered as acceptable to some but unacceptable to others?

The following examples have been chosen, first with respect to flavouring substances and secondly, with respect to the control of medicines, in order to illustrate how the Council of Europe deals with such situations when they arise.

Flavouring substances (2)

Over the years the Council of Europe has drawn up an extensive list of admissible natural sources of flavourings of plant origin. This includes edible fruits, nuts, vegetables, spices etc. from all over the world, most of which do not seem to represent any particular risk to human health.

A few, however, are known to contain toxicologically active components for which it was considered necessary to set a limit for their use in food and drink. The limits are based on information on both the amount of these components naturally present in foodstuffs and on the quantity generally used in the various countries as flavourings in the preparation of foodstuffs, as well as toxicological information where available.

The problems begin when the use of one such component is found to be significantly higher in one particular country than is usually found in the others. Pulegone, for instance, is the toxicologically active component of common or garden mint. In the United Kingdom, mint sauce is traditionally prepared to accompany roast lamb or a few leaves of this plant are used to enhance the delicate flavour of new potatoes or peas.

Mint confectionary, ranging from the famous 'After Eights' to the really strong mints is also very popular, containing levels of pulegone 10-15 times higher than that found in the usual range of foodstuffs. How then are limits set?

Bearing in mind that any limits set by the Council of Europe in this respect are in the form of recommendations to its member governments, who interpret them according to their own laws and practice in this matter, it is possible to envisage a compromise solution. Thus relatively low limits may be set for pulegone in food and drink in general, with exceptionally higher limits being permitted for use in mint confectionary. Everyone is happy, as the majority of countries use this substance very little, whereas the United Kingdom considers that the risk in using these comparatively high levels of this toxicologically active substance as both acceptable and compatible with the traditional dietary habits of its population.

Another example in this context is coumarin, the toxicologically active component of one or two other natural plant sources of flavourings. This substance is not greatly used as a flavouring in food and drink in most European countries. However, it is the essential component in relatively high quantities of a particular type of caramel much beloved by the French. Hence again an exception may be made for the limit on coumarin used in these special caramels.

A problem that has arisen fairly recently concerns the risks arising from the ingestion of smoked food. One of the reasons is that it has been clearly established that conventionally smoked food often contains certain trace amounts of carcinogenic polycyclic aromatic hydrocarbons (PAH) eg benz ( ) pyrene. Could the resulting risk be considered at all acceptable to public health? Some countries, usually not particularly avid consumers of smoked foods, feel that evidence of the very presence of proven carcinogens is sufficient to deem the risk unacceptable. Other countries, however, for whom such items might traditionally form a part of their staple diets and even upon which their livelihood might in part depend, are more willing to accept the associated risk as acceptable, at the same time welcoming recommendations to reduce as much as possible the presence of PAH resulting from the smoking method. Meanwhile, very successful and less toxic synthetic smoke flavours have been developed and the whole issue is still the subject of a somewhat lively debate.

Control of medicines
The Council of Europe has drawn up a list of medicines available on prescription only (3) in various of its member countries. The decision to control the use of a medicine by putting it on prescription is usually due to one or more reasons such as it might cause addiction, be liable to abuse, have particular toxic side effects, etc. However, the absence from the Council of Europe list of a particular medicine does not necessarily imply that it is not on prescription in one or more of the member States concerned.

Most antihistamines, for example, have been available on European markets without prescriptions for a number of years now and without any evidence of serious risk to public health. In Austria, however, the risks arising from the possible side effects have hitherto been considered acceptable only if these substances are controlled by prescription. When, however, it came to deciding what attitude the Council of Europe should take towards antihistamines, Austria agreed that control by the use of special warnings might well be more effective in reducing the associated risks than prescriptions. The majority of antihistamines do not therefore appear in the Council of Europe list and special warnings have been issued instead.

The coronary vasodilator amyl nitrite is on prescription in France and Switzerland because of the associated risks of dependence and abuse. In the United Kingdom, however, although such risks are recognised, they are considered sufficiently acceptable not to merit the use of a prescription as a control, which is left to the good judgement of the pharmacist, as well as enabling angina-prone patients to obtain such medicines rapidly in an emergency. In this case the difference in national attitudes was such that a compromise was not possible, and amyl nitrite simply does not appear in the list. Each country is free to apply the measures it considers suitable for this particular substance.

In other situations where the possibility of a compromise might be envisaged within the forseeable future, the use of a 'waiting list' is invoked. Polystyrene sulfonate resin for example, is not at present on prescription in the United Kingdom as it is not considered to be liable to abuse - added to which it is apparently extremely unpleasant to take - so its control is left to the pharmacist. Other European countries feel, however, that the risk to public health is only acceptable if the substance is controlled by prescription. Thus polystyrene sulfonate resin is on the 'waiting list' pending new developments.

One final word on the subject of clinical trials. It is generally acknowledged that these are necessary to determine both its efficacy and the side effects so that the risk/benefit of a new medicine might be determined before it may be allowed on the market.

A special group was set up within the Council of Europe to define the problems of clinical pharmacology with a view to harmonising the national procedures for clinical trials at European level. This also fitted in very well with current trends concerning the mutual recognition of data, good laboratory, practice etc., and the need to avoid duplication of the same trials in different countries.

However, those involved in this study came very rapidly to the conclusion that as things currently stood it was well nigh impossible to draw up common recommendations due to the very widely differing national attitudes towards the conduct and control of clinical trials. (For example, in the United Kingdom, the definition of 'clinical trial' does not include healthy volunteers.) The study nevertheless continued but resulted in a report of a purely advisory nature taking into account the different national situations.

Conclusions

This essentially pragmatic approach by the Council of Europe allows it considerable flexibility in dealing with situations about which not all countries see eye to eye. The fact that it has no legislative powers in this respect might generally be considered as an advantage, in addition to which any recommendations are readily modifiable in the light of new developments arising at a future date.

The principles described here have also been applied with some measure of success by the Council of Europe in its work on the safety evaluation of cosmetic ingredients (4) and plastics food packaging components (5) not to mention in its guidelines on the registration of new pesticide products (6), in which flexibility and dialogue are the watchwords. However, all that is another story which I won't go into now....

References

1. More information about the Council of Europe and its work in consumer health protection is given in the booklet:
    a. 'Partial Agreement activities in the social and public health field - 1982-1983' ref.P-SG (83) 5
    b. A list of reports, recommendations and other documents published over the years is given in doc.
    P- SG (82) 21
2. a. 'Flavouring substances and natural sources of flavourings' (1981) Bilingual 3rd edition
    b. 'Flavouring substances not fully evaluated' (Doc. P- SG (81) 26)

3. Resolution AP (82) 2 on medicines available on prescription only.
4. 'Cosmetic products and their ingredients' 1978. (NB this first edition is currently being revised)
5. 'Substances used in plastics materials coming into contact with food' (1982) 2nd edition.
6. 'Pesticides' (1981) 5th edition.

Note: All these publications, except for 2 (a) are available free of charge upon request to:
    Partial Agreement Division,
    Council of Europe,
    BP 431 R6,
    67006 STRASBOURG CEDEX,
    Tel. (88) 61 49 61.
    Telex 870943

17
'Scaling' human effects from physico-chemical hazards

A J JOUHAR

Introduction
There are two complementary approaches to assembling data in preparation for construction of a model for 'scaling' human hazards.

The first involves numerical assessments of risk based on the effects from established hazardous chemicals or by extrapolation from experimental data; and the second requires consideration of disease processes, with particular reference to their individual and societal impact and their probable relationship to causative agents.

The latter approach has the added benefit of being likely to fit better with eventual prospective use of the model for a novel chemical where one has only the animal data indicating dose-response relationships and target organ/systems, and one is extrapolating to humans. Further, this approach facilitates consideration of 'scaling' of human effects, irrespective of the class or use of the causative chemical

The operation of a physico-chemical agent results in a human health hazard with a probability (ie risk) of occurrence. With materials for which a cause-effect relationship is not certain, there is also a probability to be assigned on the magnitude of this uncertainty.

Chemicals and human ill-health
Acute accidental high exposure to chemicals may result in acute damage or disease (including 'immediate' death); and there may be chronic effects, both as primary or as secondary phenomena. Consideration must be given to this as well as to effects of 'chronic' low-level exposure to chemicals.

Also, it is necessary to look at pharmacological as well as toxicological effects (both non-neoplastic and neoplastic), in all cases with the intention of identifying the functional impact on target organs/systems. In addition, psycho-pharmacological and behavioural effects must be borne in mind.

Although the manifestations of human ill-health are so varied - as seen from the International Classification of Diseases, Injuries and Causes of Death, the range of effects is much less varied and is well encapsulated by the classical pathology terms: congenital, traumatic, inflammatory and neoplastic.

Whatever the class of effect (be it immediate or remote), their impact on physical and psychological performance affects not only the individual (through impairment of life quality, life expectancy and/or loss of earning capacity), but also the individual's family and indeed society as a whole. These interactions are shown in the Figure.

DAMAGE
(immediate or remote)

congenital
traumatic
inflammatory
neoplastic

PHYSICAL   PSYCHOLOGICAL

FAMILY EFFECT

LOSS OF   LOSS OF
EARNING   CAPACITY LIFE EXPECTANCY

SOCIETAL EFFECT

Figure

In each case one sees a functional impact on motor, sensory and psychological parameters which usually results in temporary or long-lasting disability and may or may not result in premature death. Thus, apart from shortening life 'quantity', any disability must be seen as impairing life 'quality'.

The concept of 'scaling'
These concepts make it possible to countenance 'scaling' of the human impact of health hazards, especially those resulting from the operation of physical or chemical agents. Moreover, where a cause-effect relationship is not established, the probability that such an effect exists could be used to modify the 'scaling' process.

1. Physical effects
Although these are structural, the practical effect in all cases is an alteration of function - as with loss of a limb, the development of chronic respiratory disease, neurological damage and so on.

If societal agreement could be reached, it would be reasonable to assign numerical values to these functional losses - such as a percentage of 'whole' function. This is, in a way, done already, by injury and insurance policies and by the Courts, the 'scaling' being by assigning monetary values according to the part of the body damaged. However, the 'price of a life' is not a good 'scaling' method.

2. Psychological effects
The psychological effects of damage almost certainly flow from physical effects but may arise solely from fear of a possible effect where the latent period is long; and they may be reinforced by the psychological reactions of the family.

Psychological effects also are taken into account by the Courts, through making awards for suffering and distress.

3. Loss of life quality
Only the individual can perceive his/her life quality and this perception will depend very much on the pre-existing psychological state of the individual.

121

With both psychological effects and loss of life quality, quantification is less easy, but nominal scaling ought to be possible.

4. Loss of earning capacity

Not all physical or psychological effects of damage to health result in a loss of earning capacity, nor is the duration of loss of such capacity necessarily the same as that for the effects of damage.

Clearly, premature death causes premature and total loss of earning capacity; moreover, lost earning capacity has far-reaching consequences in that society and the individual's family also are affected. Importantly, percentage quantification of lost earning capacity is not too difficult.

5. Loss of life expectancy

This is the only true quantitative factor which can be calculated actuarially, either when death has occurred or prospectively but on an empirical basis according to the disease under consideration. Clearly, early death also results in lost earning capacity and has family and societal sequelae.

6. Family and societal effects

Physical and psychological effects on the individual are likely to result in some effect on the family, both directly and through their sequel of possible lost earning capacity.

The direct effects can be seen mainly in additional psychological effects in the rest of the family with additional work-load and diversion of care and attention from other members of the family.

Societal effects mainly reflect the impact on the family - though the load on the State as a result of disability needs to be taken into account.

Proposals for 'scoring'

A useful starting point is to review the 'International Classification of Diseases, Injuries and Causes of Death' and to select those found to occur frequently (by comparison of mortality statistics) - irrespective of whether they may on occasion be chemically induced - in order to review prognosis after diagnosis. In addition, many of the conditions could be concatenated according to the above-mentioned aspects of human impact.

Data on frequency of diagnosis, frequency of medical consultation and hospitalization exist and need to be included in the disease-by-disease review. Thus, it should be possible to calculate mean age at diagnosis, mean life expectancy for the disease groups in question and, in many cases, mean duration of hospitalization.

This will give nominal data for reduction in life expectancy. It may be that any shortening which is less than two standard deviations from mean life expectancy should be ignored, since this amount of 'shortening' is by definition, within the bounds of normality.

These data then could form bases for scaling.

Since people react differently to physical damage, perhaps the only way of 'scoring' is to make value-judgements on the basis of severity of the physical damage and/or its permanence (though permanence can be taken into account by factoring for duration).

For lost earning capacity, 'scoring' ought to be relatively easy (though perhaps a factor for the effect of lost level of expectation needs to be included).

By using historical data for 'sickness duration' according to diagnosis, loss of earning capacity can be evaluated; also, it can be factored for certain conditions according to the techniques used in assessing disability awards.

With family effects, the age of onset of damage to the individual is material, but can be taken into account through factoring for duration; however, it is necessary perhaps to include something for the 'family commitment' (eg the average family unit being the individual plus spouse plus 2.2 children) and perhaps the State commitment through likely disability or other pensions.

In general terms, the societal effect of damage to the individual is measurable from lost earning capacity and from assessment of any State commitment; this in result needs not to be factored separately.

Examples

The main factors to include in 'scaling' are:

      physical effects
      psychological effects (including life quality)
      loss of earning capacity
      family and societal effects
      reduction in life expectancy

By assuming a life-span of 68.5 years (to simplify the mathematics), each individual has a span of 25 000 days. By assigning a maximum of 1 for each day's duration of effect for each of the first four factors, a total score of 100 000 is obtained. All four factors score where life expectancy has been reduced. Alternatively, and since the mean life expectancy is greater than 68.5 years, a 'score' of 8 could be assigned for each day of life for each factor, thus totalling 1 million for maximum. This might have an added advantage in that value-judgements can be applied to the 'day-score' of 8 multiples of eighths. Such 'scoring' would come into operation with 'death at birth' (eg an abortion) or birth with massive congential deformities (eg the 'thalidomide child'). Other hazards (ie conditions) would score less that 100 000 (or 1 million).

Example 1

Occupational cancer - diagnosed at 58 and death at 60

- loss of life expectancy 13 years
- suffering 2 years
- incapacitated last 0.5 years

physical	-	2 x 365 x 0.4=	292
psychological	-	2 x 365 x 0.8=	584
lost earning	-	0.5 x 365 x 1=	182
family/society	-	2 x 365 x 0.8=	584
life expectancy	-	13 x 365 x 4 x 1	18 980
			-----
			20 622

Example 2

Chronic bronchitis - diagnosed at 35 and death at 70
- loss of life expectancy 0 years
- suffering 25 years
- incapacitated last 5 years

physical	-	25 x 365 x 0.5=	4562
psychological	-	25 x 365 x 0.4=	3650
lost earning	-	5 x 365 x 1.0=	1825
family/society	-	25 x 365 x 0.2=	1825
life expectancy	-		0
			-----
			11 862

Example 3

Brain damage from vaccination at 2 years of age; currently at home; life expectancy of 20 years
- loss of life expectancy 55 years
- suffering 18 years
- incapacitated

physical	-	18 x 365 x 0.9=	5913
psychological	-	18 x 365 x 0.2=	1314
lost earning	-	=	0
family/society	-	18 x 365 x 0.9=	5913
life expectancy	-	55 x 365 x 4 x 1—	80 300
			-----
			93 440

Example 4

Blinded in an industrial accident at 22
- no loss of life expectancy
- suffering 51 years
- incapacitated only for 5 years

physical	-	51 x 365 x 0.2=	3723
psychological	-	51 x 365 x 0.2=	3723
lost earning	-	5 x 365 x 1=	1825
family/society	-	51 x 365 x 0.1=	1861
life expectancy	-	=	0
			-----
			11 132

'Scaled' in this sort of way, one can differentiate between the human impact of a variety of disparate conditions. In the examples given (which are purely illustrative), blinding in early adulthood is of similar impact to developing disabling chronic bronchitis later in life. A late-developing occupational cancer has a somewhat greater impact, and the occurrence of brain damage associated with vaccination is a major occurence.

Second, the importance of hazards which have been identified by experimentaion and extrapolation can be kept in better perspective. It is not enough to say that a chemical has been shown to produce cancer in the rat; it is essential to try to assess the human impact of such carcinogenesis.

Last, the addition of a ranking order to human impact from a variety of conditions, to the current procedures of identifying hazards and extrapolating risk levels, should refine the process of risk assessment.

Societal acceptance of such concepts and agreement on value-judgements in some areas will be necessary: however, these problems are, it is believed, capable of being overcome.

Index

Advisory Committee on Major
  Hazards   17
Advisory Committee on Toxic
  Substances   96
Ageing   27-29
Allergy   12, 80-81
Animal carcinogens   55-63, 73-76,
  105, 113-116
    genotoxic   58-59
    non-genotoxic   59-61
    pseudocarcinogenicity   61-63
Asbestos   9, 11, 34, 96

Biological considerations   78-82

Cancer   13, 45-46, 69, 73-76, 96,100,
  114f, 123
Carcinogen Panel (UK)   46
Cardiovascular disease   48-50
Chemicals   vii, 11, 34-35, 41-47, 53,
  73-76, 78-82, 95, 97, 99f
Chemicals Industries Association
  (CIA)   95, 99-101
Coal dust   31-33
Committee on Safety of
  Medicines   49
Congress (US)   3, 70, 111, 114
Consumers   11-16, 51-54
Cosmetics   51-52
Council of Europe   117-119

Department of Energy (US)   18
Diethystilbestrol (DES)   6, 11, 13
Drugs, monitoring of   14,
  48-50,   118-119

EEC   51-54
Electronics industries   9
Emergencies   9, 11-12, 17f
Employees, occupational
  risks of   30-36, 78-82, 94-107,
  121-125

Epidemiology   97-99, 104

Food Additive Amendments
  (Delaney Clause)   112, 115-116
Food and Drug Act   v
  Food and Drug Administration
  (US)   6, 49, 70
Food, risks from   6, 12, 52-53, 111-
  118

Gregson report   94

Handler, Philip   43, 111
Hazard range   19f
Health and Safety Executive
  (UK)   6, 18, 25, 95, 99
Health risks 3f, 30-36, 41-47, 78-82
Hypertension   48-49

Industry, risk management in
  17-26, 30-36, 94-107
Institute of Occupational
  Medicine   32
International Agency for Cancer
  Research   105

Local Authorities   18
Log-probit method   69

Malthus, Thomas   5
Maslow, Abraham   29

National Academy of Sciences
  (US)   45, 111-112
National Cancer Institute (US)   46
National Coal Board   31-33
National Health Service   28, 96
Nuclear power   6, 13, 33
Nuclear Regulatory Commission   6

Occupational hazards - see
  Employees
Office of Population Censuses and
  Surveys (OPCS)   42f, 46
Opren   11, 14

Parliament, Acts of   v, 9, 44
Pesticides   12, 14-15
Pharmaceutical companies   49-50
Physico-chemical hazards   120-125
Pneumonconiosis   31-33
Polychlorinated biphynyls
  (PCBs)   7
Polyvinyl chloride (PVC)   73-77, 95
Popper, Karl   14
Pott, Percival   68
Public awareness of risk   v, 3-10, 13,
  67f, 89f
Public health policy   10f

Risk
  'acceptable'   viii, 67-72
  decision-making   3-10
  quantifying   5f, 18f, 30f, 67-72,
    120-125
  'zero'   3, 20, 67f
Robens Report   95

'Scaling' effects   120-125
Statistical techniques   69f

Third World   12
Trades Unions   96f

Vinyl chloride monomer
  (VCM)   73-77, 95-96

Yalow, Rosalyn   7